1987

Medical Ethics:
Common Ground for Understanding

Kevin D. O'Rourke, OP, JCD
Dennis Brodeur, PhD

The Catholic Health Association of the United States
St. Louis, MO 63134-0889

Library of Congress Cataloging-in-Publication Data

O'Rourke, Kevin D.
  Medical ethics.

  Includes index.
  1. Medical ethics. 2. Physicians—Professional ethics. 3. Medical
ethics—Case studies. I. Brodeur, Dennis. II. Title.
R724.075   1985   174'.2   85-21349
ISBN 0-87125-109-4

Copyright © 1986
by
The Catholic Health Association of the United States
4455 Woodson Road
St. Louis, MO 63134

We wish to acknowledge the patient and continuing help of June Granville, our friend and assistant. Because she has been such an integral person in the work of the Center for Health Care Ethics, and because she also has labored to produce these essays, to her we dedicate this volume.

Table of Contents

Acknowledgments

The best part of our six year effort to build an education and research program in health care ethics has been the support and challenge offered by our students and colleagues at SLUMC. While the support of officials of all the schools and hospitals affiliated or associated with SLUMC has been outstanding, we do wish to thank explicitly George E. Thoma, MD, whose idea it was to institute the Center for Health Care Ethics to serve the entire medical center; Thomas C. Dolan, PhD, director of the Center for Health Services Education and Research at SLUMC; William Stoneman, III, MD, dean of the medical school of Saint Louis University; and Richard Stensrud, MHA, chief executive officer of Saint Louis University Hospitals.

Introduction

   Medical Ethics: Common Ground for Understanding is a collection of essays written for students and professors at the St. Louis University Medical Center (SLUMC) as one element of an educational program. The essays were written monthly by the staff of the Center for Health Care Ethics, often in response to questions of medical ethics being discussed in the media. Over the years, however, other individuals, schools, and hospitals have requested copies of the essays and at present over 300 other institutions use them in their education programs. At the suggestion of several of our students and colleagues, we are making the essays available to an even larger audience.

   Though sponsored by the Society of Jesus (the Jesuits) and thus a Catholic institution, SLUMC attracts faculty and students from many different ethnic and religious backgrounds. The people of SLUMC are a pluralistic community similar to our society at large. Hence these essays, while not in conflict with Catholic teaching, are written for a pluralistic community.

   Because the essays are designed for a pluralistic audience does not imply that they are without logical foundation or principle. Medical ethics founded on personal opinion, emotional reactions, or on an erroneous concept of the human person does more harm than good. Rather, these essays are based upon two objective realities: (1) the functions that human persons have in common; and (2) the goals of medicine as evidenced in the physician-patient relationship. Hence, in the essays one will find frequent reference to the physiological, psychological, social, and spiritual functions of the human person. Moreover, it will become clear that while health care in the strict sense is concerned with only the first two functions, it must respect the other two. The equality of persons in the physician-patient relationship and the desire to heal physiological and psychological functions while respecting social and spiritual values will also be a theme. Though these essays are directed toward a pluralistic community, we draw upon a very definite concept of the human person and some precise values and goals of the healing relationship that we believe have brought out the best in people in the health care professions over the centuries.

While this collection is not presented as a textbook or a model for logical progression in the science of medical ethics, we hope that it will stimulate critical thinking, prompt discussion, foster a reasoned understanding of objective principles and, above all, help people actively involved in health care or serving on ethics committees to ask the right questions when faced with ethical issues.

The essays are gathered in three general sections with no reference to the time at which they were written. Part one contains those essays examining the concept of medical ethics for a pluralistic society and expressing some thoughts on the physician as ethicist. While we center upon physicians as the audience and subject of the essays, we include implicitly other health care professionals. Thus, what is predicated of or directed to physicians applies *mutatis mutandis* to nurses, hospital administrators, people in allied health care professions, trustees, and those in any way associated with health care.

Part two considers some general principles of medical ethics. The consideration of principles is not taxonomic; rather, we present some of the more important principles, seeking to ground medical ethics in values and objective reality as opposed to opinion and erroneous concepts of the human person.

Part three considers cases that have been prominent in the media as well as critiques of articles that have appeared in medical journals. While we do not always seek to solve the cases in question because information sufficient for an informed ethical decision is seldom presented in the media, we do seek to present the principles that should be utilized in answering similar questions that might arise in the course of offering health care. In response to the journal articles, we seek to consider the assumptions upon which they are based, to analyze the reasoning of the articles, and to state the implications of the conclusions when these are ethically significant for health care professionals.

During the past six years the type of ethical issue facing health care professionals has changed. While the ethical questions in the past were directed toward medical procedures (for example, informed consent, transplantation of organs, and allowing patients to die), today and in the immediate future the more prominent ethical issues in health care will be social issues: why and how to care for the poor; how to preserve quality of care in the face of government controls and fiscal constraints; how to preserve the values of medicine in the face of efforts to commercialize health care; how to choose which health care services will be offered from the many valuable services available. Though the issues change, the principles and values used in ethical decision making should remain the same. Hence, while some of the cases and issues presented may seem dated, we believe a reasoned analysis of these cases will be helpful to meet the ethical issues of the future.

Medical Ethics and

Professional Responsibility

Medical Ethics: 1
A Common Understanding

Many individuals and professional organizations maintain that ethics committees must be formed in hospitals in order to help answer the questions arising from advanced technology and increased recognition of patients' rights. Even if the committees are confined to a role of educational activities and not given the power to make ethical decisions for others, a practical question arises: What principles will the committee use when deliberating about ethical issues or when trying to formulate policy to be presented to the administration for approval? Drawing together ten people with ten different ethical perspectives might bring chaos rather than consensus. Is there a common understanding of medical ethics that will enable people on ethics committees to function cooperatively and intelligently despite different professions, backgrounds and religious persuasions?

Principles

Medical ethics arises from the relationship between a patient and a physician. The patient goes to a physician seeking health. Health, in this limited sense, is well-being of physiological and psychological functions. Health is of great value for the patient, but it is not the only value. The patient has values associated with social or spiritual functions as well.

The physician enters the relationship promising to help the patient achieve health. This promise implies two presuppositions: (1) the physician will strive for competency in the field of medicine; and (2) the physician promises to respect the patient as a person. Hence, in addition to the value of health in a limited sense, the other values (social and spiritual) the patient might have will be respected. Thus the physician agrees to respect the patient's quest for health in the wider sense of the term. This latter respect for social and spiritual aspects arises from the fact that the physician respects the patient as an equal. Although the patient is subordinate or unequal to the physician in medical skill and knowledge, he or she deserves respect as a person of equal worth insofar as the other values of life are concerned.

Often there will be no conflict between the patient's health values and social and spiritual values. In most circumstances patients look upon healing (a physiological or psychological value) as a necessary means for achieving other values in life (social and spiritual). Thus, in most cases, difficult ethical decisions will not be in question because no choice between conflicting values is necessary. Rather, these routine cases call only for protection of the patient's basic rights as a human being (e.g., the right to be informed, the right to maintain one's reputation).

But in some cases there will be a conflict between maintaining or restoring health (achieving psychological or physiological values) and achieving social or spiritual values. For example, an aging patient suffering from a terminal illness may decide that he or she would be better off spiritually if life-prolonging therapy were withdrawn and death allowed to ensue. A person might believe that divine law prohibits the use of blood transfusions even if they would prolong life. In cases of this nature the conflict must be settled by treatment that respects the patient's values. The ethical basis for the patient's right to choose the type of treatment is the fact that as a human being the patient is equal to the physician. When entering the healing relationship the patient does not surrender personal responsibility for determining which values are more important in a given situation.

In like manner the physician does not surrender his or her value system when entering the healing relationship. Thus there may be difficult ethical decisions for physicians to make as well; for example, is it contrary to my value system to allow a patient to die when I know life could be prolonged? Should I operate on the person who refuses blood transfusion knowing there is increased danger of death? Hence the medical relationship seeks to achieve health but does not posit health as the ultimate human value for patient or physician.

Discussion

The goal of healing the patient in accord with his or her value system serves as the touchstone of ethical medical practice in particular and of health care in general. Of course, other factors should be considered in medical and health care; for example, economic and societal factors enter into the offering of medical and health care. These economic and social factors are especially prominent today with the national focus on cost effectiveness, competition and reducing use of health care facilities. Although these economic and social factors must be considered by the ethical physician or hospital administrator, they must never be allowed to dominate the practice of medical care or health care. If they do, then a perversion of values occurs, and physicians and other health care professionals betray the trust of patients and their own integrity. Resisting the pressure to make economic or societal factors the basis for decision making will be difficult for ethics committees as well as for physicians and other health care professionals.

From the nature of the healing relationship and the presuppositions mentioned above, the general principle of medical ethics can be deduced. For example, in order to enable patients to express their value systems and to ensure they are treated as equals, informed consent is required; informed consent gives rise to the principle that health care professionals should tell the truth; because the patient's reputation is of great value, the principle of confidentiality is posited.

Although these and other principles of medical ethics are deduced from the nature of the physician-patient relationship, they should not be applied as though they were straitjackets determining every particular decision. In practice, two patients may be treated differently because each might have a different value system. Thus medical ethics is not relativistic or circumstantial because it does have valid general principles. But it is flexible because these general principles must be applied to individual patients who have different needs and value systems. Facing death, one person might choose life-prolonging therapy; another might choose only pain-relieving therapy.

Conclusion

Ethics committees can be helpful if the people serving on them have a common understanding of the nature of medical ethics. Judging from the literature on the subject, however, ethics committees often seem to be promoted as a means of defusing moral responsibility or of avoiding malpractice litigation or of removing the anguish from difficult ethical decisions. There is no way to make difficult ethical decisions easy. People serving on ethics committees would do well to ponder constantly the question: Do we have a common understanding of medical ethics?

Can We Agree?

Medical history shows that in every age, medical practice has been embroiled not only in scientific controversies, but also in ethical ones. The introduction of vaccination, the use of quinine, the administration of anesthesia, performing heart transplants, and defining death through lack of brain activity all produced serious ethical controversies. Many of these ethical issues continue to this day and are hotly debated. The unfortunate side effect of ethical debate is that people often become discouraged with reaching an agreement. Thus they separate into diverse groups and ultimately converse only with people with whom they agree. Health care professionals often wonder why such sharp differences exist in the realm of medical ethics.

Principles

Ethical questions are inevitably controversial for various reasons, including the following:

1. Ethical questions are complex, involving many different factors; it is thus possible to get different results by emphasizing different aspects of a problem. Thus in the abortion issue, for instance, one group emphasizes the rights of the mother and the other group emphasizes the rights of the unborn child, and little dialogue results.

2. Ethics deals with profound and mysterious issues of human life such that our knowledge of values involved is incomplete and always open to further study.

3. Ethical matters cannot be completely universalized into rules because they involve the individual and individual situations, so there is always a difficulty in applying general rules to concrete cases. Thus ethics is not relativistic because all human beings have much in common. But applying principles to individual cases is more than a mathematical procedure.

4. Ethics treats questions not only of fact but also of value. Values influence both our thought and our feeling and will. They involve an essential element of subjectivity as well as an objective foundation in human experience.

5. Ethical decisions not only affect abstract questions, but also directly change our personal lives. Because such change is painful, it is difficult not to be prejudiced in ethical judgment, since "no person is a good judge in his or her own case." Usually people try to defend their prior ethical positions rather than subject them to criticism.

6. Ethical perceptions depend on our concrete experience, and all persons or groups have their own history and special culture which profoundly influence their ethical outlook. Thus we are intimately involved in our ethical viewpoints.

7. Fundamental to all particular ethical judgments is the religion or its equivalent philosophy of life with its value systems to which the individual or group consciously or unconsciously adheres.

8. Besides the difficulties that arise from our human finitude are the difficulties that have their origin in what is called human sinfulness, which darkens our understanding and distorts our motivation. Whether this sinfulness is the result of human history embodied in social structures or of our own individual contribution to this human condition is in a sense immaterial. It is present in our lives, whether we look on it as primarily social or primarily personal.

Discussion

In view of these difficulties, how are we to develop a satisfactory and mature approach to ethical controversies in medical discussion? A hint of an answer can be derived from the psychological studies of Jean Piaget and Lawrence Kohlberg, which have shown that in most groups of adults there are persons at different levels of development in ethical thinking, corresponding to the phases through which a child must pass to full moral maturity. These phases can be summarized in three main levels:

1.The small child tends to make decisions on the basis of the immediate consequences of an action (i.e., rewards and punishments).

2. The growing child begins to make decisions more and more on the basis of social approval of parents or peers. Conformity to group norms becomes paramount, and satisfactions can be delayed and suffering incurred to achieve approval of others.

3. Moral maturity is marked by an increasing internalization and independence of such moral judgment. Decisions are now made on the basis of personal standards, and the standards of society become subject to criticism. The adult acts primarily for self-approval, even at the cost of disapproval by the group.

Most ethical controversies seem to be carried on largely at the second level. The debaters each proceed on the assumption that the value system of their group, whether it be that of a social class, a professional elite, or a church, is self-evident, and they make little or no effort to understand the viewpoint of opponents who live within other, competing value systems. This mindset has been demonstrated by various groups within the field of health care as they disagree over ethical issues; however, it is also demonstrated by health care professionals as a group as they disagree with other groups in society over values. For example, associations representing health care professionals seem continually at odds with associations representing people interested in reducing health care costs.

In the United States the four main value systems involved in most public debates are humanism, Judaism, Catholicism, and Protestantism with their many subsystems. Because each of these groups rests its arguments on assumptions the others do not share, public controversies on medical-moral matters such as abortion or therapy for the dying tend to end in stalemate. However, with patience and fairness it may sometimes be possible to pursue a question to the third and mature level of ethical thinking, in which it becomes possible to subject even these assumptions to examination, reinterpretation, and, we hope, eventual ecumenical convergence. Ethical discourse of this nature requires patience, understanding, and generosity.

The Values Inherent   3
in Medical Care

Values influence—and in many cases determine—human behavior; they give direction and meaning not only to individual actions but also to our personalities. What values are associated with health care? Are any values so closely associated with medical care that to neglect them would frustrate the effort to offer that care? In order to study these questions adequately, we shall consider the concepts of health, human function, and health care.

Principles

Health and health care are interdependent; hence, to understand the values associated with health care, one must possess a clear notion of human health. Ask the physician, nurse, or hospital administrator, "What is health?" and you are liable to receive a blank look in reply. Henrik Blum concludes a searching analysis of the concept of health with the brief formula, "Health is the state of being in which an individual does the best with the capacities he has, and acts in ways that maximize his system." Because a human being is an organism, it is an open system. Hence, in maintaining balance or homeostasis a person is continually relating to the environment. For our purposes, then, we conceive of health as optimal human functioning, which implies not only an internal harmony and consistency of function, but also the capacity of the organism to maintain itself in its environment.

What is conveyed by the term *human function?* Human beings are born with the need to eat; because we feel hunger (the need for nutrition in order to survive), we perform the function of eating. We have a capacity for knowledge; because we feel a need for truth in order to understand and fulfill our purpose in life, we perform the function of learning. It is widely acknowledged that there are four categories of human needs and corresponding functions: (1) biological or physiological;

(2) psychological; (3) social; and (4) spiritual or creative.

Given these basic needs and functions, it is extremely important to discern how they are related, since this relationship will provide a blueprint for the quest for health and the limits of medical care. Is one function more important than another? If so, it will contribute more to health. Are the relationships among the various functions cooperative or competitive? Can one function be sacrificed for another without impairing the individual's health?

These four functions are not stories in a building, one on top of the other, but rather interrelated dimensions of human activity. Just as the length, height, and depth of a cube can be distinguished conceptually for sake of study, but not separated in reality, so the four functions of the human act are interconnected. Every truly human act involves all four functions. A human spiritual act, whether it be the creative act of a scientist or the loving act of a parent, at the same time involves a biological, psychological, and social function. True, one type of function will predominate in a human act, but all types will be present.

The task of the creative function is to integrate the biological, psychological, and social functions. Thus creative functions are the deepest, most central, and most complex. At the same time, however, these activities are rooted in and dependent on the other functions in a network of interrelations. One cannot think unless one's brain is physiologically sound. Moreover, each function is to a certain extent autonomous, structurally and functionally differentiated, so that when help in restoring function is needed, each function is served by a different discipline. To restore the physiological function of bones, for instance, an orthopedist is called; for psychological function, a psychologist or psychiatrist is needed; for the social function, a social counselor or lawyer is required; for the creative-spiritual function, a teacher or spiritual director is called for.

The ultimate goal of health care then is an optimally functioning human person. Notice that this concept is richer and more complex than the ultimate goal put forward for health care by many ethicists: the autonomy of the person.[1]

Discussion

Clearly, physicians and all other medical care professionals must be concerned proximately and primarily with healing the physiological and psychological functions. However, their efforts at restoring these functions must be performed with the awareness of the interrelatedness of all human functions. Thus, the ultimate goal of health care must be health in the fuller sense: the coordinated functioning of all human powers. Physicians who do not realize the interrelatedness of all human functions might think they have the right to make all decisions for the patient; health planning might be directed only to the betterment of physiological functions without regard for their relation to psychological, social, or spiritual functions.

Even though patients present themselves in a wounded state of health, as a result of which they have lost some degree of self-determination, the patient's power to make his or her own decisions must be respected by the physician and all other persons in health care. Because of the good in question, and because there is a need to respect the patient's spiritual integrity, a specific type of relationship arises between the physician and the patient, known familiarly as the professional relationship. The heart of this relationship is an avowal (*professio*) that one person is willing to help another person attain an important human good while at the same time respecting that person's personal worth and dignity. Given the service value in the relationship between the professional and the person in need of help, it is evident that the relationship must be built on trust. This is especially true in medicine, where the patient's vulnerability is multidimensional and the patient-physician relationship is intrinsically imbalanced.

If our brief account of the values inherent in the medical relationship is accurate, then it is clear why profit cannot be the primary basis of any profession, but must be considered a secondary and highly variable feature. Traditionally, a principle fundamental to all professions has been that the professional must be ready to give services free to those who are in need but cannot pay. Indeed, official codes of medical ethics usually state that fees should be adjusted to the ability of the patient to pay.

In view of the foregoing analysis of health, medical care, and the physician-patient relationship, the following value statements are normative for individuals and corporations involved in health care:

1. Those offering medical care must remember and respect the worth and higher functions of the individual: this implies something more than mere "autonomy";
2. The overriding purpose of medical care must be a desire to serve those whose physiological or psychological health is impaired in order to enable them to lead a better life;
3. The patient-physician relationship must be permeated by trust;
4. Medical care should not be considered a commodity, something to be bought or sold in a market system, because it is a precious and vital good to which no price can be attached and because it is prerequisite to the attainment of other human goods as well as to the pursuit of a meaningful life.

---

1. Charles J. Dougherty, *Ideal Fact and Medicine*. (New York: University Press of America, 1985), p. 66 ff.

The Assumptions   4

of Physician-Patient Relationships

Economics, the delivery of health care, rights and justice, cost, technology, and a host of other issues confront American society at a time of tremendous socioeconomic and institutional change in health care. Some of the problems are new, but many are not. An article by Sanford Marcus in the *New England Journal of Medicine* addresses one topic: trade unions for physicians, as a paramount concern for the medical profession.[1] Perhaps physicians' salaries are threatened by the changes in the health care field, and perhaps it is necessary for physicians to band together to protect themselves from the unjust "paymasters" of today's health care system. The point can be argued. But the real difficulty of Marcus' argument is not the notion of physician unions, but the underlying assumptions about health care.

Principles

Marcus' claim is that physicians have been worried about a threat from the left—a growing notion that there is a right to health care requiring a national health insurance. Government intrusion into the physician-patient relationship will make the medical profession civil servants. This concern blinds them to the fact that entrepreneurial growth from the right can irrevocably change medicine, leaving the physician compromised in terms of autonomy and financial compensation. The new "paymasters," as he refers to them, prefer to deal with physicians independently while subtly undermining the basic principles of medicine. Physicians, in turn, are expected to lose graciously and accept the new ways of corporate medicine. Their other choice, according to Marcus, is to cling tenaciously to the traditional ethics and principles of medicine and experience inevitable death.

Physicians must ask what they want. First, Marcus contends, they want to be a part of the healing profession;

second, they want to be compensated fairly "somewhere on a scale between that of a day laborer and that of Michael Jackson." In order to realize these goals, physicians must learn to negotiate and find adequate legal representation, not available through the American Medical Association because of antitrust laws, and fight for the right to do whatever is necessary for patient care, quality assurance, and financial reimbursement. If unions are established, physicians may have to strike to gain their purposes. A strike would not eliminate emergency care, and ultimately the strike weapon would ensure quality care for the patient and adequate compensation for the physicians. The union's time has come, Marcus asserts.

Marcus continues the discussion of service-oriented unions and strikes. The article asks: Are unions the best representation model for nurses and physicians? How does one handle the troubling economic issues in medicine? What social policy should govern relationships? But most troubling are the assumptions that underlie Marcus' argument.

Discussion

Four of his assumptions must be examined. The first is that the patient-physician relationship is completely closed. No one else, and certainly no institution or government, has any right to be a part of this relationship. In addition, it is the autonomous power of the physician that will protect this value. Second, there is a direct correlation between the physician's ability to unionize and the assurance of quality care for the patient. Strikes disrupt the product base of the owners in order to adversely affect profits and thereby win concessions. When patients are the product base for the health care institution, it is hard to imagine that they will benefit. In addition, the altruism required to give up something for oneself in order to benefit someone else is not in great supply in modern times. The third assumption is that the health care institution is simply a warehouse for the physicians' tools and health care facility. Quite the contrary, the institution is considered a moral agent with responsibilities to the patient. The final assumption in the article is that the greatest promotion and advance of people's health is accomplished through the practice of medicine.

If Marcus used a different set of assumptions there might be very different conclusions. The first assumption is that the patient-physician relationship is crucial, but that no matter how excellent the decision made in this relationship, it is always done within a societal framework. It is the responsibility of *both* the physician and the patient to consider cost, benefit, and other social values. Patients and physicians must be aware of medical costs and make intelligent choices. Ironically, the past period of reimbursement based on actual cost brought about entrepreneurial involvement, government "intrusion," and business coalitions. Physicians, patients, and institutions must look at their own behavior to understand the reasons behind some of the recent developments in the health care "industry." Physicians, because of the privileged relationship, have an important role to play in resolving economic issues through research, peer review, and public policy input.

Physicians, like any other group of people have rights to congregate to promote their own purposes. No one would deny them adequate compensation, but compensation is secondary on a priority list. One could question how unions fit into the broad definition of professional associations. Physicians are not plumbers, automobile workers, or custodians. Their right to form unions and to strike is tempered by the fact that the heart of their professional identity is service to those in need.

Medicine works only where there is a cooperative and consensual relationship between patients and professionals. Patients have multiple needs that require a team approach. Physicians may head the team, but they are not the total team. Health care institutions exist to serve the multiple needs of the community in which they exist. Adversarial relationships between the institution and the physician will not advance patients' needs. Even if the structure of medicine changes, the centrality of the patient and the need for consensual work remains vital.

Finally, medical treatment is not necessarily the primary promoter of health in this country. Numerous studies show the importance of primary care and preventive measures, better nutrition, sanitary living conditions, no smoking, and less alcohol are necessary ways to improve health and extend the life span. If physicians are truly concerned about better health, their involvement in these areas is crucial. Patients will lose not because the physician has become the employee, but because there is no one who advocates healthful living.

Conclusion

Marcus is correct that recent changes in the ownership and organization of health care institutions have affected the physician. These problems must be addressed. However, different assumptions than this lead to a very different kind of argument, a different conclusion, and better health for one's patients.

1. Sanford Marcus, "Trade Unionism for Doctors," *New England Journal of Medicine* 311(1984): 1508-1511.

Ethical Norms for Medicine   5
in the United States

Who formulates the ethical norms for medicine and health care in the United States? Perhaps some people would respond to this question by saying that the American Medical Association formulates the ethical norms for medicine and health care. Others might say that ethical norms are formulated by the philosophers or theologians, and still others might say that, for them, their churches formulate the significant ethical norms. Some truth exists in each of these answers, but a more important source of ethical norms for medicine and health care in the United States is the federal government. Because the presence of the federal government in the field of ethics is novel and even revolutionary, it merits further comment. This chapter offers a few thoughts and comments about the history of this presence and the work of various federal commissions in the field of medical ethics.

History

In the late 1960s and early 1970s, Congress became uneasy, in fact disturbed, about the implications of scientific progress. Revolutionary advances in science and technology were predicted, for example, genetic engineering and DNA splicing, and it was feared that these advances might have damaging effects on individuals and society. Fresh in everyone's mind was the experience with atomic power during World War II. The strong belief of Americans that scientific progress always leads to a better life had been destroyed at Nagasaki and Hiroshima. At the same time, public outrage arose over some scientific research projects that had violated the human rights of some individuals. For example, a study was made public in which aborted fetuses were decapitated in order to perform pharmaceutical tests. Moreover, the Tuskeegee Syphilis study, which withheld from some poor black men afflicted with syphilis the cure for this disease, was revealed. Hence, due to the general apprehension about revolutionary scientific developments and the sharp public reaction to specific abuses in the area of research, Congress in July 1974 brought into being The Commission for the Protection of Human Subjects of Biomedical and Behavioral Research (CPHS). As its name indicates, the mandate for this commission was to set ethical guidelines for research projects involving human beings, especially those whose rights might be violated. When the life of this commission ceased, the Secretary of the Department of Health, Education, and Welfare appointed an ethical advisory board (EAB) in the spring of 1978 to continue the study of ethical issues and public policy. This advisory board was superseded by another group created by Congress on Nov. 9, 1978, called The President's Commission for the Study of Ethical Problems in Medicine and Biomedical and Behavioral Research (PCEMR).

Accomplishments

The productivity of the three above-mentioned federal commissions has been impressive. The CPHS published more than ten studies in its four-year life on such subjects as research on fetuses, children, prisoners, and the mentally infirm; it also studied psychosurgery, put forth ethical guidelines for delivery of health care by government agencies, and set forth standards for institutional review boards (IRB). In the Belmont report, the CPHS sought to synthesize the ethical principles it had used in its studies. The EAB, because of its short existence, studied only one ethical problem at length, that of in vitro fertilization. The PCEMR was commissioned by Congress to consider many ethical issues, such as brain death, availability of health services, and testing in regard to genetic disease. It has published ten reports, ranging from brain death to access to health care. These reports are marked by sound scholarship and a desire to improve health care in the United States.

Discussion

No attempt will be made here to evaluate any of the particular documents put out by the above-mentioned federal commissions, but the following general comments are offered:

1. The very fact that Congress recognized the need for ethical norms in the field of research and therapy is a step forward. For the most part, the norms set forth by the commissions are useful and protect the rights of scientists and physicians as well as subjects and patients.

2. The norms formulated by the commissions are designed with our pluralistic society in mind. Thus they seek to enunciate what most scientists, politicians, and religious thinkers will agree on. Although they do not state it explicitly, they tend to avoid controversy; hence some of the more difficult and important ethical issues are not considered; for example, the value of human life, the moment at which human life begins, and whether all have a right to health care.

3. Although some of the more important norms concerning physician-patient relationships are considered, for example, informed consent and justice in selection of research subjects, there is not sufficient consideration of the following pressing ethical questions: Should all feasible care be financed publicly? What are the goals for our national health programs? How can we determine priorities in health care? Are health care professions too powerful or self-serving?

4. The basis on which these ethical statements are formulated is seldom the nature of the human being, the covenant between physician and patient, the just society, or religious teaching. Rather, the basis is usually what is culturally acceptable. Deciding ethical responsibilities upon what is culturally acceptable is dangerous because it justifies whatever is popular. Ethicists should continually question and evaluate what is culturally acceptable, judging it on more fundamental values.

Conclusion

In sum, the deliberations of the federal commissions have been worthwhile in that they have brought to our attention the need for ethical norms in the field of research and therapy. But because the agencies avoid some of the more important questions as they concentrate on expressing consensus, it is clear that more rigorous thinking must be applied to the modern ethical issues in medicine, research, and health care.

The Ethical Physician 6

Self-understanding is the beginning of wisdom, but in order for it to be possible, one must have the benefit of honest reactions from other people. Otherwise, no opportunity exists for objective evaluation and testing of one's subjective thoughts and attitudes.

What is true of individuals is true of a profession as well. Unless the members of a profession receive honest and objective information from people outside the profession, there is little hope for healthy and effective self-understanding. Over the past few years, the profession of medicine has received candid and worthwhile evaluations in regard to its ethical perspectives and standards from scholars outside the profession.[1] Some of these evaluations may be summarized as follows:

1. Most physicians have a "strong sense of vocation" rooted in the original priestly character of medicine and reinforced in American culture by the religious stress on vocation. Yet this religious motivation has been covered over: "The vast growth of science and technology in the four hundred years since Luther has obscured the specifically religious conception of most vocations. The physician seldom speaks of God anymore when discussing his concern for the patient. Yet he still finds satisfaction in measuring up to personal standards."[2]

2. To be effective, physicians maintain they must be motivated and competent and must show concern for the patient. An important component of motivation is physicians' sense of specific competence; that is, they have an important and well-defined service to offer. Much of physicians' personal satisfaction in their work depends on this sense of competence. Most physicians believe they must "care for the whole patient," but only a minority of physicians have a well-developed social conscience.

3. Physicians tend to think pragmatically, so their basic attitude can be characterized thus: "The physician sees himself as a professionally competent person who is in a social position to apply scientific knowledge and to exercise impartial control over the situation in order to achieve the rational goal of curing or helping a sick patient. The patient's part of the job is to trust the doctor and cooperate with him."[3]

4. Furthermore, physicians on the whole do not regard themselves as research scientists, but rather as applied scientists, and they do not clearly experience a dichotomy between the scientific and the humanistic or affective aspects of medicine. Their satisfactions are not theoretical but pragmatic.

5. Physicians take much satisfaction in their professional position as a mark of achievement. This sense of achievement is more important for physicians than monetary rewards, which they do not like to think of as a primary motivation. Moreover, although physicians gain some satisfaction from scientific interest in their work, they gain more from therapeutic results. An important element of satisfaction or dissatisfaction is found in the sense of consistency between personal and professional ethics. Thus physicians do seem to have a common sense of ethical purpose.

Discussion

Some possible ethical biases that medical professionals should be aware of and that medical education should strive to balance if the medical profession is to make good ethical judgments are as follows:

1. On the whole, physicians continue to exhibit the dualistic balance between the scientific and the humanistic. The balance is constantly imperiled, however, by the fact that their scientific training is explicit, detailed, and specialized, while their humanistic and moral training is left largely to example and symbols transmitted to them without explicit reflection or criticism. Physicians thus assume that although science is exact, ethical discourse is vague, subjective, and a matter of opinion. On the one hand, this assumption leads to a kind of moral skepticism; on the other, to a dogmatic rigidity, since no method of dialogue or research for critical consensus is available.

2. Physicians tend "to take a pragmatic view whereby what is most valued is an immediate, practical solution."[4] In ethical matters, this pragmatism may lead physicians to act so that (1) they will not be made to feel guilty if an action is taken

against their professional or personal standards; (2) they will not seem inhuman toward the patient; (3) they will not go beyond the limits of the patient to wider social problems; and (4) they may be more concerned about the law than about ethics.

3. Because physicians' motivation is so bound up with their sense of vocation, autonomy, and competence, they resent interference in their own decisions. They believe that only physicians are in the position to make medical-ethical judgments and that they can be relied on to be decent and humane in these decisions. This attitude may lead to deeply felt but simplistic attitudes toward ethical questions.[5]

4. Physicians often resent that so much responsibility is laid on their shoulders. They cannot understand why a wider sociological, religious, psychological, or interrelational view should be their responsibility. Physicians believe such concerns are someone else's business.

Conclusion

These attitudes undoubtedly are the result of the medical professional's need to live by a clear motivation, with manageable responsibilities, and to have sufficient freedom for action and personal judgment. If they result in a closed attitude that renders the physician incapable of learning from others or sharing in a team effort to improve ethical treatment of health problems on a social scale, however, they are harmful biases that may lead to gravely mistaken ethical judgment.

1. Ford, Amasa, *The Doctor's Perspective: Physicians View Their Practice* (Cleveland: Case Western Reserve University Press, 1967).
2. Ford, p. 140.
3. Ford, p. 144.
4. Eliot Freidson, *Profession of Medicine, A Study of the Sociology of Applied Knowledge* (New York: Dodd Mead, 1971), p. 147.
5. Wendy Carlton, *In Our Professional Opinion* (South Bend: University of Notre Dame Press, 1979), p. 173.

A retired physician and medical educator, Ludwig W. Eichna, MD, went back to medical school in order to experience the realities of present-day medical education. In 1980 he recounted his experiences in the *New England Journal of Medicine* and listed eight principles that he believed should underlie a needed and thorough renewal of medical education.[1] The eighth and last principle is that "the profession of medicine demands at all levels, specifically including that of medical students, the highest ethical conduct." In discussing this principle, Eichna offers three statements that demand comment because they manifest a concept of ethics that is inadequate and that underlies the problem of poor ethical formation in medical schools.

Statement 1: "Ethics is not really taught by lecture or seminars...one teaches medical ethics by living it and expressing it in daily actions." In keeping with many scientists, Eichna presents an anti-intellectual view of ethics. Science and truth are one thing; ethics and personal opinion are another, might be the way Eichna's position could be expressed. On the contrary, ethics is just as "scientific" as biology or mathematics if we understand that the material we are studying in ethics, namely, human actions, is infinitely variable and subject to innumerable modifications because of human freedom. Because of its scientific nature and content matter, it is absolutely necessary that ethics be taught in lectures and seminars in medical schools so that health care professionals will develop a well-grounded, deliberate, and rational method of reaching ethical decisions.

In considering cases drawn from realistic medical situations portraying people who have experienced these situations, ethics courses should offer problem-solving exercises that Eichna says are lacking in contemporary medical education. With principles drawn from the profession of medicine itself (not excluding, but not depending on, the tenets of religious faith), ethical presentation of this nature provides an objective basis for medical personnel to make ethical decisions. Although no one denies that ethical conduct requires "living it and expressing it daily in actions," this overly practical view of ethics is simply inadequate because it leads to subjective decision making. Perhaps the reason that another retired medical educator, Robert Ebert, MD, recently wondered whether medical schools are creating an environment "which permits success to become a more coveted commodity than ethical conduct" is the fact that the scientific presentation of ethics was long ruled out of medical school.[2]

   Statement 2: "Schools contribute to the teaching of bad medical ethics through indoctrinating students in the 'me first' state of mind...and by allowing students to look upon patients as impersonal beings that exist for the students' own development." In contrast, Eichna believes that students must be taught to care for the whole patient and that "the patient comes first." It is the second part of the statement that gives us pause. Eichna, looking for a reason to substantiate a better ethical outlook toward patients, becomes too altruistic. "The patient comes first" ethic represents an exaggerated and unrealistic ethical norm for the profession of medicine. If we build medical ethics on the principle of "the patient comes first," we are putting the physicians and other health care professionals in a dangerous situation where they are disposed to ignore their own needs and human development under the guise of serving others. This attitude has most likely been destructive of personal and family life for many physicians.

   Given that medical students must have the opportunity to work with patients, what principle should be communicated to students in order to help them develop ethical attitudes and conduct toward patients? The principle on which ethical patient care must be based is the contract that a physician makes with a patient. The physician, as a professional, assures that he or she will help heal the patient. Usually the physician focuses on physiological or psychological care, but these are only partial elements in the process of healing. The spiritual and social elements must be considered as well. Thus the physician is committed to a concern for the whole person simply because such concern is necessary for healing.

   Statement 3. "Society is creating an environment that teaches students bad medical ethics...with compulsive attention to the cost of medical care." Eichna's overall assessment of the role of economics in ethical medical care seems to lack social perspective. Although he does not state it explicitly, he seems to maintain that the ethics and economics of medicine can be separated. This conviction stems from the idea that ethics is merely a personal affair and has nothing to do with public policy, an idea held by many politicians as well as scientists. Actually, if the practice of medicine is to be ethical, physicians must be concerned about public policies, especially public policies that control economic resources. When a physician treats a patient, ethical concerns do not allow that he or she treat that patient as if no one else in the world exists or as if the needs of other people are unimportant. Indeed, the important ethical problems in regard to the profession of medicine today are not centered in the physician-patient relationship. Rather, they are centered in the physician-patient-society relationship. To put it another way, the principles for deciding ethical issues in regard to informed consent, prolonging life, or truth telling are rather clear. The truly difficult questions are: What percentage of the gross national product should be spent on health care? What aspects of health care should be developed and what should be eliminated? Do people with unhealthy habits have a right to care from tax monies? Can society impose restraints on people in order to improve the health of others? The ethics of medicine, then, is a social as well as a personal science.

Conclusion

In sum, Eichna's call for more emphasis on ethical education in medical schools and in the medical profession is laudable, and the renewal is overdue. But the concept of ethics used must be more scientific, more realistic, and more socially oriented than the one with which he seems to be working.

1. Ludwig W. Eichna, "Medical Education 1975-1979: A Student's Perspective," *New England Journal of Medicine* 303(1980): 727.
2. Robert Ebert, "A Fierce Race Called Medical Education," *The New York Times,* (July 9, 1980): 27.

Ethical Issues in   8
a Pluralistic Society

      In 1973 the Supreme Court of the United States ruled that abortion of an unborn fetus at any time during pregnancy is not to be prohibited by law. Contrary to the opinion of many, this decision did not make abortion legal for the first time in the United States. Before this decision, it had been legal in most states when pregnancy had resulted from rape or incest, and in some few states it was legal without restriction. Yet as anyone who has observed the scene in America will realize, the abortion decision of the Supreme Court caused dissension, division, and even hatred among the American people. Other medical ethical issues of similar importance and concern are waiting in the wings. For example: Given the increasing cost of health care, will we set an age limit for certain treatments and thus shorten the lives of many? Realizing that some people do not care for their health, will we limit the care offered to repeated drug and ethanol addicts? When and how will we allow genetic experimentation on human beings? If these medical-ethical issues are not settled in a more expeditious manner than the abortion question, we set the stage for continued strife, become immobilized to handle other issues, and encourage a subtle disintegration of common values. Our purpose in this essay is not to solve any of these medical-ethical issues, but rather to suggest a methodology for working toward political and legal policies in regard to these ethical issues in a pluralistic society.

Principles

      In a pluralistic society, many groups with different value systems come together to strive for important common goals. In the United States the important goals that unite the society are in the *Preamble* to the Constitution. These goals are in themselves a value system; together in this society we seek justice, unity, civil peace, security, prosperity, and personal liberty for ourselves and our posterity. In addition to stating consensus about important goals, people in a pluralistic society realize there are other important values, call them second-level values, about which some agreement must be reached. In order to foster agreement on second-level values, the legislature is formed; in order to protect the central and second-level values, the judiciary is formed. But both legislature and judiciary are at the service of values, whether central or second-level, not vice versa. Fundamentally then, the various legislatures and courts in the United States are value measured and receive their power and efficacy when they are faithful to human values of the commonwealth.

But reaching consensus on the statement and protection of second-level human values is not an easy process. In unimportant value issues, each person or group can be free to follow a personal value system as long as others are not injured. But in those areas where lack of consensus would lead to a gradual or sudden destruction of the ability to seek and protect the central values of society, there must be some consensus. This consensus must be more than the lowest common denominator, or otherwise we are likely to frustrate the purpose for which we come together. Thus in a pluralistic society, we must reason toward consensus and hold the central value as the measure of our consensus, not the values of any individual group.

All groups should be allowed to enter into the dialogue that will develop consensus concerning second-level values. Thus religious groups have as much right to participate in the dialogue as any other group. Our statement of central goals ensures that no religious group will be given favor, however. Moreover, it implies that religious groups must enter the dialogue on the grounds of reason, not on the grounds of faith. Thus, because something is approved or forbidden in the Torah, the Gospels, or the Koran, does not mean that for that reason it should be approved or forbidden in our pluralistic society. Only if values proper to a particular religion can be presented "scientifically," persuasively and reasonably should they be approved as part of the consensus concerning secondary values. If a religion teaches that rape is wrong, a believer cannot insist on religious grounds alone that laws against rape are mandatory. In order to seek laws against rape, one must prove that rape destroys the meaning of human sexuality and places violence at the center of a relationship that should be founded on love and consent.

Discussion

As even the most secular or legal experts will note, the Supreme Court reached decisions in the abortion cases that were not founded on any consensus or attempt at consensus in the public forum. Hence, through what one member of the Court called "an act of raw judicial power," the Court sought to impose consensus upon the nation. Thus a legal decision was made that was not based on value consensus. As one writer observed in the *Wall Street Journal* ten years after abortion was legalized: "A wide range of scholars holding both pro and anti-abortion beliefs quickly pointed out the numerous problems with *Roe v. Wade.* These included mistakes in history, science, and law. But the essential difficulty was, as it remains today, that *Roe v. Wade* imposed on the nation a view of the abortion issue lacking constitutional warrant."[1]

But could the Supreme Court have acted otherwise? It seems that courts and legislatures are not capable alone of developing consensus on these difficult medical-ethical questions. Where would they go to find consensus on the issues in question? Was there a forum for developing consensus concerning the following vital questions: When does human life begin? Should the right to life of a woman ever supersede that of the fetus? There were religious views of these questions and views that were supported by science and reason, but there was no forum for people to discuss them and reach some consensus.

Is the situation any better today? One federal commission has served as a forum for such value determination. The President's Commission for the Study of Ethical Problems in Medicine and Biomedical and Behavioral Research (PCEMR) has already published some significant studies (see p. 19), but the commission must be continued and enlarged so that it represents a wider cross-section of society. Voluntary commissions of this nature would help at the state level, too. Many state legislative acts amount to value statements concerning issues on which there is not yet consensus. For example, living will legislation implies that physicians will not treat patients inhumanely. We are not naive enough to believe that development of consensus will ever be an orderly and perfectly rational process, but, on the other hand, legal and judicial policies used in the past to develop consensus concerning medical-ethical issues are simply no longer effective.

1. *Wall Street Journal* (1/22/83): 4.

How Health Care   9
Becomes a Business

Well over 100 years ago, the perceptive Frenchman, Alexis de Tocqueville, wrote: "Americans have a passion for health, well-being and equality." Perhaps if he were viewing the scene in the United States today he would say, "Americans have a passion for health and well-being at the lowest possible price." The concern about the cost of health care that pervades the thinking of policymakers in the United States in our day is not in itself detrimental or ill-conceived. Use of human resources and material goods in a manner that benefits all members of society is of ethical as well as economic concern. If the cost of health care continues to escalate, many people, especially the poor, will not be able to afford such care. Moreover, other needs of society, such as education and care for the mentally ill, will not receive enough support if more and more funds are devoted to health care. Hence, our concern is not about the effort to contain rising costs in health care, but that, in so doing, the nature of health care will be changed from a profession to a business. To put it another way, by reason of the methods employed in the effort to contain costs, health care is being changed from an humanitarian to an exclusively economic endeavor.

Principles

Consider, for example, that the language people use to describe their occupations is often an accurate indication of the way they conceive of themselves and their occupations. Consider the way the emphasis on economic factors has changed the language of health care. Whereas we used to speak about the *profession* of medicine or health care, we now speak about the health care *industry*. Whereas we used to speak about patients, we now speak about *consumers.* Physicians, nurses, and hospital personnel have become *providers.* Health care professionals used to offer health care;

they now *deliver* health care. Medicine and medical procedures and practices used to be evaluated in regard to their power to alleviate pain or to heal; now *cost effectiveness* is all important and the ultimate evaluation of medical practice is whether it enables people to become, once again, *productive members of society.* The list of words could be multiplied, but the implication is clear. The total effect of this terminology is to make medical care a commodity—something akin to wheat, sand irons, or popcorn; thus the "laws" of economics become the touchstone for medicine.

Not only the language used to describe medical care but also the subjects discussed at national meetings indicate how extensive is the takeover by economics as the "final solution." Study the programs of the annual meetings of the American Hospital Association, American Medical Association, and the American College of Hospital Administrators to see how many topics concern legal or economic issues as opposed to humanitarian patient care. Finally, the emphasis on economics even leads some health care professionals to use wealth as a measuring stick for their professional and personal accomplishments; the amount of money they earn, the number of homes they possess or how many successful real estate investments they make being for some the criteria that gives them worth and meaning.

Discussion

Looking on the profession of medicine and health care exclusively as a business destroys its essential meaning. Medicine and health care are founded on the realization that human beings have a set of needs that are interactive; these needs usually are enumerated as physiological, psychological, social, and spiritual. Health care professionals serve people directly in regard to their physiological and psychological needs; however, the needs are so intertwined and interactive that health care professionals also influence indirectly, and sometimes directly, a person's social and spiritual needs. Thus the health care professional does not work with a biological specimen or with an isolated part of the human entity; he or she works with an integrative sensing, feeling, thinking, loving human being.

To help a person integrate his or her needs, to help a person maintain or regain health and well-being requires in the character of the physician such talents as wisdom, compassion, and human concern. The health care professional who is truly humanitarian says to the patient: "I shall try to heal you at every level of your being and help you become a whole person. In so doing, I shall respect your integrity as a person and treat you as an equal." The professional promises knowledge, skill, and, above all, concern for the person who comes for help. In the health care profession, concern for the patient is not something "nice" or extraneous, not something added to avoid malpractice litigation. Rather, it is an integral element in the science and art of the healing profession. Moreover, the concerned and perceptive health care professional realizes that many of the really important questions (e.g., Is there a God? Does life have meaning? Will I exist after death?) surface only at the time of serious illness. The competent and compassionate health care professional is concerned that patients be able to address these questions and live with the uncertainty they generate.

Is this an idealistic view of health care? Yes, it is. But unless people have ideals that are challenging and altruistic, eventually they will lose interest in what they are doing and very often become cynical or depressed. Health care professionals are especially endangered by this syndrome of cynicism and depression because they experience and share intense human suffering, suffering that often does not seem to have any meaning. They often give time and energy to people who do not seem to have self-respect or a desire to care for themselves. Unless their ideals enable them to transcend the suffering, sorrow and squalor of the hour and day, there is danger that they will be overpowered by their experience or seek relief in frenetic activity.

Conclusion

If there is any truth in the concept of health care described briefly above, then the implications of allowing economic factors to dominate thinking and planning in health care are evident. Qualities such as wisdom, compassion, human concern, and service do not translate into economic values. If the present trend to use economic terminology and economic evaluative criteria continues, the realities these words represent as well as the words themselves will be removed from the profession of health care. Thus one of the professions that for centuries has called forth the very best in human beings will become just another fungible element in the rapacious diversion called the world of business.

Economics and Health Care: 10
The Dominating Values

There are many signs that the profession of health care is losing its sense of direction. The American Hospital Association sponsors a "comprehensive conference on hospice care," but the purpose of hospice care, namely, to enable dying people to prepare spiritually for the experience of death, is not mentioned. Rather, the agenda is devoted to reimbursement, financial management, payment, and insurance issues. The Society of Hospital Planners holds its annual meeting, and quality patient care is not discussed. Rather, the topics considered are the competitive edge, commercial strategy, aggressive marketing, and pricing strategies. Looking through the material announcing various seminars and workshops, one is hard pressed to find anything that even mentions the purpose of health care, namely, the beneficial development of a human person by ministering to physiological or psychological needs. Nor does one discern any appreciation of health care as a profession, that is, an occupation that must stress caring and compassionate attitudes and values in order to be successful. However, any number of conferences offer to explain diversification, corporate revision, and cost per case management. Last year, writing in the *New England Journal of Medicine,* John F. Burnum depicted the effect of this overriding commercial emphasis in health care on the fictitious Doctor Z.[1] Although whimsical, the article is tragic as well. Doctor Z is stripped of his hospital privileges because "he refused to accept the guiding principles of the new medicine: that the encounter with the patient is accurately and completely defined by a disease diagnosis and that for every disease there is corresponding technological treatment." Lest you sympathize with Dr. Z, realize he is the cause of his own downfall because "he was never able to think of medicine as an industry and view hospitals as a business...he clings to the archaic belief that medicine is an ethical rather than a commercial enterprise."

Principle

Undoubtedly many people will respond to the commercialization of health care by citing the need for economy, cost effectiveness, and surplus in the contemporary health care environment. The argument is often phrased thusly: "If there is no profit, there will be no hospitals and health care." Every perceptive person would agree with this statement. Moreover, they would agree that it is wise to discuss marketing, diversification, and anything else that will contribute to economic responsibility. While discussing these items, however, unless people continually remind themselves of the purpose of health care, they will be inclined to make money the dominating motive of the health care system in the United States. History and our own experience demonstrate that the unsubordinated pursuit of profit brings out the worst in people. Such attitudes as avarice, selfishness, and exploitation are more likely to dominate the pursuit of profit than are those person-centered attitudes that bespeak compassion and care. Care for the sick, whether they be rich or poor, requires skill, dedication, and generosity of spirit. The qualities and attitudes that are required to care effectively for people are not the qualities and attitudes needed to make a profit in business.

Hence, the question facing us is which attitudes, values, and characteristics are going to dominate and influence the provision of health care: those which bespeak compassion and respect for the person who is in need of help, or those which bespeak competitive pursuit of financial effectiveness? The growing tendency for the values and attitudes of commerce to dominate the provision of health care is found in the phrase "the health care industry." Anyone who truly appraises health care as an industry as opposed to a profession is on the way to accepting the values of competitive commerce as the dominating force in health care. To appraise health care as a profession, on the other hand, does not imply that one approves inefficient or wasteful business procedures. It does mean, however, that one places, as the ultimate norm for both patient care and business procedures, such values and attitudes as competence, humility, commitment, and compassion. Managers, accountants, planners and marketing researchers must be well aware of the values and attitudes that should dominate their activities as they employ their knowledge and skills to improve the efficiency and effectiveness of those directly involved in the profession of health care.

Discussion

Unfortunately, the nominal leadership in the profession of health care does not recognize the importance of the question: Which values will dominate the profession of health care in the future? When evaluating diagnosis-related groups, for example, the American Medical Association bases most of its considerations and observations on financial concern for physicians. At a recent conference on care for the poor, when "cream skimming" by for-profit hospitals was declared detrimental to teaching and public hospitals, a leader of the American Hospital Association could only respond, "Tension has always been there, but the association has to be an industrywide association." When the leaders of the health care profession refuse to acknowledge their responsibility and opportunity to care for the poor, then health care is indeed in danger of becoming an industry.

What can individuals and institutions do to foster and develop health care as a profession? First of all, health care professionals should watch their language, avoiding the jargon and slogans inflicted on the health care profession by accountants and economists. Second, those planning conventions and medical meetings should include ethical issues on the agenda. Finally, and most importantly, institutions should develop and take seriously a mission statement used as the ultimate norm for every program, policy, and action. Brief and accurate, the mission statement should place the patient's health and well-being as the goal of health care and discuss the values that should dominate the pursuit of this goal. Of course, the proof of the mission statement will be in its use and application. Individuals as well as institutions may develop a mission statement. As a health care professional, how would you express your purpose? Developing a concept of purpose helps liberate one from the dehumanizing commercialism that infects so many involved in health care.

Whenever a group of people lose direction, the reasonable remnant must seek to stay on course until the others recover their senses. Despair and recrimination are not in order, but committed people must continually remember their purpose as health care professionals and their dominating values and act accordingly.

---

1. John F. Burnum. "The Unfortunate Case of Dr. Z: How to Succeed in Medical Practice in 1984," *New England Journal of Medicine* 310(1984): 729-730.

Medicine and Economics   11

The increasing cost of health care services concerns hospital administrators, physicians, planners, and third party payers. New structures and financing mechanisms to provide health care have been created within the health care profession. The hope is that these new structures will contain the rapidly increasing price of health care, help institutions maintain financial solvency, and pressure all involved to be more efficient in their use of health care services while maintaining or bettering the health care status of the public. There is a major difficulty in such a plan, however, because the aims and goals of medicine do not always match the purposes and goals of economic structures.

Principles

The starting point and central focus of health care is the idiosyncratic need experienced by a person when illness strikes. The random nature of illness and the "art" of the practice of medicine make it hard to establish fixed guidelines that are applicable to every patient and every institution. Patient benefit, expressed in the ethical principles of beneficence and do no harm, requires that physicians and all other providers attend to the needs of the patient before other considerations are allowed to affect the medical relationship. Related to this is the role of the provider as professional. Normally one defines the provider as a person who serves the needs of others through his or her acquired skills and competency. Service usually requires a certain amount of advocacy for the patient. Subsequently, the provider responds first to the needs of the patient and does not allow other financial, political, or institutional concerns to preempt this relationship.

In the larger social setting, this care is a requirement of justice. People should not be deprived of basic health care services. Unlike other justice issues, however, access to health care is not a matter of equality of opportunity, but is considered on the basis of need. Differences may exist in how many resources are consumed by one person, but the difference is not based on merit or future promise or personal financial solvency. The individual's health care problems are the basis of services delivered.

Discussion

If this were an ideal world in which no fiscal restraints existed or all social values could be realized, choices would not be necessary. But because there are limits on the amount of money that can be poured into health care (limits not yet clearly defined) and because other values and goals compete in common life, choices must be made.

Economic structures or new financial strategies have been one attempt at making choices. The assumptions are that health care should be considered like any other commodity in the free market system. This implies that consumers are in charge of the market and that their choices will dictate where and how dollars are spent. The "health care market" should then respond to consumer demand. This should create a competitive environment that will reduce the dollars spent and create new ways of delivering more affordable health care more efficiently. This would result in greater cost containment and put a stop to the rapid rate of increase in health care costs. The rise of business coalitions and various new directions in methods of payment reflect this kind of philosophy. The question is: Will it work?

Simply stated, these two sets of assumptions do not mesh. Medical care begins on the basis of need with a promise that those in need will receive care. The economic assumptions imply that some needs may not be fulfilled and that certain people will have to forego some kinds of health care.

In the past few years some institutions have been closed. Some people use alternative delivery sites; lowered costs have been realized in some instances. In 1984 the number of beds occupied and the average length of hospital stay decreased significantly. Some services, such as home health care, have increased, and more long term care beds are filled. In addition, it may be fair to say that the federal government will have "contained" its health care costs, especially under the new diagnosis-related groups system.

What is not known is whether a reduction in physician visits or hospital days means anything more than a short-term savings. What may occur in the long run is an increased number of people in poorer health. The government may have capped its Medicare costs, but that does not mean that the health status of the nation is better. Some of the excess beds in the country may be eliminated, but whether they will be eliminated in the overcrowded suburbs or the underserved urban and rural areas of America has yet to be determined. Some institutions have responded to the present economic environment and entered into new agreements with many different groups lowering some health care costs, but this has also resulted in less money available to the elderly, the poor, and the underinsured.

Conclusion

Any compromise or resolution between these two sets of assumptions must consider the primary factors that contribute to greater health status of people. More research and attention must be paid to the high-technology therapies that are truly beneficial; to the various tests and procedures that are truly helpful in making an accurate diagnosis; to the type of delivery site that best promotes the patient's values and needs. The public must assume more responsibility for personal issues of life style that affect health and become more knowledgeable about the practice of medicine so that defensive medicine is not practiced and unnecessary adversarial litigation is avoided. Providers and the public must become partners in cost-conscious choices about medical care.

In addition, some continued national discussion about the levels of services that can be judiciously rendered to all people is needed. When the value issues underlying health care are addressed, then the question of which economic strategy will best help realize the nation's health care goals can be raised. If, on the other hand, the economic questions are asked first, the values and goals of medicine will be determined in ways foreign to the profession of medicine. Choices must be made, but they will be better made from a thoughtful reflection of patient needs and values than from a concept of health as a commodity.

in Hospitals

Recently, the American Hospital Association (AHA) recommended that each hospital institute an ethics committee. Perhaps the action of the AHA is due to the study of ethics committees recently published by the President's Commission for Ethics in Medicine and Behavioral and Biomedical Research.[1] Although the commission stopped short of recommending that an ethics committee be established in each hospital, it clearly recommended that education, consultation, and review be available in each hospital for difficult decisions of patient care. The purpose of this chapter is to consider the purpose and functions of an ethics committee in hospitals and to evaluate its usefulness.

Principles

Ethics committees in hospitals received their main impetus from the decision of the New Jersey Supreme Court in the Karen Quinlan case. The court, assuming erroneously that most hospitals had ethics committees, declared that such committees rather than the courts should be involved in decisions concerning withdrawal of life-support systems. In analyzing the hospital ethics committee, the President's Commission lists six potential functions:
1. Review a case to confirm the physician's diagnosis or prognosis of a patient's condition;
2. Review decisions made by physicians or surrogates about specific treatment;
3. Make decisions about suitable treatment for incompetent patients;
4. Provide general educational programs for staff on how to identify and solve ethical issues;
5. Formulate policies to be followed by staff in certain difficult cases; and

6. Serve as consultant for physicians, patients, or their families in making specific ethical decisions.

Discussion

Clearly, the last three functions are of an educational nature and they could be carried out in regard to routine ethical issues as well as crises. The first three functions are not educational; rather, they could be termed jurisdictional powers because they bespeak a review power and, in some cases, a decision-making power. These jurisdictional powers are needed, the commission maintains, in ethical cases that involve the medical treatment of incompetent patients who are in danger of death. For example, the ethics committee with these powers might be called on to affirm or deny the medical opinions that a patient is in a coma, to make a decision about withdrawing life-support equipment, or to review the decision-making process to ensure that all concerned people were consulted.

The Quinlan court and the AHA are interested in having hospitals form ethics committees with jurisdictional powers. The main concern of the court seems to be that cases concerning treatment for incompetent moribund patients be settled in the hospitals and not referred to the courts. The main concern of the AHA seems to be that costs be controlled by removing life-support systems as soon as possible, while necessary safeguards to avoid malpractice suits are observed. Although the concerns of the court and the AHA are legitimate, there are definite difficulties that accompany giving jurisdictional power to a committee within a hospital. First, it may remove the medical and ethical decisions from the persons who are responsible for the decisions. In caring for dying people, whether competent or incompetent, physicians have the responsibility to make ethical decisions based on medical facts. This responsibility cannot be given to other persons nor to a committee. The patient, or the patient's family if the patient is incompetent, also has ethical responsibilities that should not be delegated.

Second, giving review or decision-making power to the ethics committee may dilute the ethical decision-making process rather than improve it by weakening concern for the good of the patient. Everybody's business is nobody's business. In referring ethical decisions to a committee, there is a built-in potential for enervating the decision-making process by emphasizing secondary factors, such as economic concerns.

Third, the introduction of a review system for treatment of patients at the time of death could lead to a wider review system of all cases with cost-control implications. The use of high technology in diagnosing patients' conditions could be subject to these committees also. In sum, then, it does not seem that placing the review or decision-making powers in the hands of the ethics committee will lead to better treatment of people in danger of death.

On the other hand, it seems the ethics committee would be able to fulfill its purpose through educational functions alone. Formal health care education in the recent past has not prepared people for competent ethical decision making, and it does not look as if the situation will improve in the immediate future. The solution to this perceived lack of preparation, however, is not to put ethical decision making in the hands of a few. Rather, there should be "on-the-job" opportunities for health care professionals to assimilate the general and specific knowledge pertinent to ethical decision making. This can be done in a number of ways; through workshops, case studies, and consultation in individual cases, health care professionals can acquire the knowledge necessary for ethical decision making.

In addition, knowledge may be enhanced if the ethics committee outlines policies, to be approved and put into effect through the usual administrative process, for specific ethical problems. For example, several hospitals are formulating policies on withholding cardiopulmonary resuscitation. These policies do not remove the ethical responsibilities from the concerned persons; rather, they ensure more effective personal decision making because they set the limits within which such ethical decisions will be made.

Conclusion

Decisions concerning the care of people who are near death, whether they are old or newborn, involve many medical and ethical difficulties. There is no way to ensure that such decisions will be easy, but we can ensure that insofar as humanly possible such decisions will be well-informed and responsible and made with the benefit of the patient as the foremost and determining factor. We submit that given the history of health care and medicine, and given the tendency to impersonal decision making by committee process, all concerned will be better served if the responsibility for decision making rests with physicians, patients, and patients' families, rather than with an ethics committee.

1. President's Commission for Ethics in Medicine and Behavioral and Biomedical Research. *Deciding to Forego Life-Sustaining Treatment* (Washington, DC: U.S. Government Printing Office, March 1983).

General Principles

of Medical Ethics

Informed Consent 13

Informed consent is back in the news. An issue of the *New England Journal of Medicine* contains two articles that indicate that this most important ethical and legal norm ensuring patient's rights is not well observed.[1]

The first article demonstrates that patients often do not understand clearly the content of the informed consent form.

> Within one day of signing consent forms for chemotherapy, radiation therapy, or surgery, 200 cancer patients completed a test of their recall of the material in the consent explanation and filled out a questionnaire regarding their opinions of its purpose, content, and implications. Only 60 percent understood the purpose and nature of the procedure, and only 55 percent correctly listed even one major risk or complication... only 40 percent had read the form carefully... and only 27 percent could name one alternative treatment.

The second article, using two standard tests, analyzes the readability of consent forms from five representative hospitals. The conclusion is that "the readability of all five were approximately equivalent to that of material intended for upper division undergraduates or graduate students. Four of the five forms were written at the level of a scientific journal, and the fifth at the level of a specialized academic magazine."

In both of the articles the authors call for a revision of the forms used for informed consent and the process by which the information in the form is communicated to the patient. Our purpose is not to confirm nor to deny the conclusions in the above-mentioned articles; they speak for themselves. They also offer, however, an opportunity to review some thoughts about informed consent and to discuss why it is necessary for ethical decision making.

Principles

The ethical and legal requirements for informed consent are (1) information, (2) comprehension, and (3) voluntariness.

1. The specific *information* that should be provided for the patient concerns the purpose of the procedure, anticipated risks and benefits, alternative procedures, and hoped-for results. Information should never be withheld for the purpose of eliciting consent, and truthful answers should always be given to direct questions. If a research project is in question, then information may be withheld provided the subject is informed that some information will not be revealed until the research is completed and that no direct harm results from withholding the information.

2. *Comprehension* of the conveyed knowledge is a requirement more complex than it might at first seem. Because subjects' capability to understand varies so greatly, the material must be adapted to the subjects' capacities. Health care professionals are responsible for ascertaining that the subject has comprehended the information, especially if the risk is serious. If the patient cannot comprehend, then some third party, usually a family member but sometimes a person appointed by the court, should be asked to act in the patient's best interest. Some have maintained that comprehension of difficult medical terms is not possible for the ordinary person, but research has shown that persons unfamiliar with medical terms can understand and retain explanations about medical procedures if the explanations are well-planned and given in plain language.[2]

3. *Voluntariness* implies that the person understands the situation clearly and that no coercion nor undue influence is exercised by the health care professional. However, it is often difficult to determine where justifiable persuasion ends and undue influence begins. The health care professional who believes that some particular treatment is better for the patient should state his or her conviction but should also explain clearly the reason for this opinion. Voluntariness does not imply that the patient will be free from all pressure or persuasion in a given circumstance. For example, a person

with an inflamed appendix is limited insofar as freedom of choice is concerned. But voluntariness does imply that, over and above the limitations arising from the circumstances, no external coercion or moral manipulation is present.

Discussion

Some think that informed consent is required only for research protocols or for experimental procedures. Actually, informed consent is required for any action that would affect a person's physiological, psychological, or moral integrity. Why is informed consent so important? Does it merely help avoid malpractice, or does it fulfill an important human need?

Respect for persons, one of the most basic ethical principles, is carried out in practice through informed consent. The patient's right to informed consent arises from the conviction that human beings are responsible for their own actions and their own destinies. They must be treated as equals and allowed to make the important decisions of life for themselves whenever possible. Only in this way will they be able to reach their full potential as human beings. Although the health care professional offers help to the patient, in return the health care professional is not given the right to make decisions for the patient nor to manipulate the patient. Health care professionals will dispose for the total and integrative betterment of the human beings whom they serve only if they are careful in observing the requirements of informed consent.

---

1. B. Cassileth, "Informed Consent—Why Are Its Goals Imperfectly Realized," *New England Journal of Medicine* 302(1980): 896; and T. Grunder, "On Readability of Surgical Consent Forms," *New England Journal of Medicine* 302(1980): 900.
2. William Woodward, "Informed Consent of Volunteers: A Direct Measurement of Comprehension and Retention of Information," *Clinical Research*, 27(Sept. 1979): 248.

Proxy Consent: 14
Deciding for Others

Four recent, well-publicized, and highly controverted legal decisions determining medical treatment (Quinlan, Saikewicz, Spring, and Fox) are concerned with the notion of proxy consent. These cases provide an occasion to review the ethical norms for this form of consent and to comment briefly on the aforementioned decisions.

Whenever possible, informed consent on the part of the subject is ethically and legally necessary for every medical treatment and research project. Sometimes, however, the subject is not able to give consent. For example, an aged person in a coma, an infant, or a fetus cannot perform the rational act necessary for informed consent even though he or she may require some medical treatment. In such cases, another person is called on to offer consent: this is called proxy or vicarious consent.

Principles

Although proxy consent is often identified with informed consent, the two are quite different. Proxy consent is not a subspecie of informed consent; rather, it is a substitute for informed consent and is sought when acquiring informed consent is impossible. For the ethical and legal use of proxy consent, two conditions must be present: (1) the patient or research subject cannot offer informed consent; and (2) the person offering the consent must determine what the incompetent person would have decided were he or she able to make the ethical decision. This second condition is difficult to ascertain and may be subject to dispute.

Decisions of proxy consent should be made in view of the good of the individual patient, not for the higher good of society, nor for a class good, because this would amount to manipulation of the person. When deciding on the treatment for a comatose person dying of cancer, for example, the proxy must seek to determine what the patient would decide if able to make the decision. What would benefit people other than the patient should not be considered unless it can be assumed reasonably that this would have been the consideration of the patient. Hence, parents of a neonate with serious birth anomalies may not say, "Let the baby die; he will be a burden to us." Rather, they must make a decision in accord with the good of the child, weighing especially the fact that in most cases we judge life to be a gift worth preserving, even if living may involve working with handicaps or infirmities. Because some parents abuse their rights to decide for their children, there is a trend to question the rights of parents to make proxy judgments and to insist on a better system of checks and balances than exists presently.

Discussion

Because of the nature of a proxy judgment, the person given the right to make such a judgment for another should be one who knows the person well and who has a loving concern for his or her well-being. Usually, then, the person who is presumed to have a legal and ethical right to make a proxy judgment is the parent, spouse, or next of kin; however, others, such as physicians and ethical or spiritual counselors, should be consulted.

The presumption that a parent, spouse, or relative will judge rightly is especially strong because of the bond of love that unites such a person to the patient, but of course this is not an absolute presumption. It may yield to a contrary fact. Thus, if the person who has the right to make this decision decides on something that does not seem to be in accord with the good of the patient, other responsible people may challenge the decision of the proxy and even bring the matter before the civil authority. Physicians, nurses, and hospital administrators who determine with good reason that the proxy is not acting in accord with the patient's best interests have the ethical, and sometimes legal, obligation to intervene and ask the court to limit or abrogate the rights of the parent or relative by appointing another person to act as proxy. The aforementioned legal decisions are examples of the court's intervening in the treatment of a patient in this manner. Unfortunately, in the Saikewicz, Spring, and Fox decisions, the courts determined that only the legal authority can act as proxy for removing life-sustaining equipment in life or death situations. These decisions arrogate to public authority matters that belong in the private and personal domain and show a general lack of trust for loved ones to interpret the wishes of a comatose and, in these cases, dying person.

Conclusion

These decisions were reached because the courts based their thinking on the notion that preserving life is an absolute good, and thus the courts "have no choice but to intervene and examine each case on an individual patient by patient basis."[1] Although preserving life is a highly valued good, and although when doubt exists the proxy should decide in favor of prolonging life, in some circumstances the proxy may determine ethically to allow a person to die. For example, when prolonging life would not serve any human purpose or would impose an intolerable burden on the patient, the decision to withhold or remove life-supporting therapy may be made as long as the normal care due a sick person is maintained. Thus it seems that a more nuanced ethical evaluation would have kept all of these cases out of court in the first place. Be that as it may, the usurpation by the courts of ethical decision making can be viewed only with great alarm.

---

1. *Eichner v Dillon*, 426 NY State 2d., 517, 550 (App. Div. 1980).

Telling the Truth to Patients   15

"What to tell the patient" has been considered one of the more difficult and delicate ethical questions for health care professionals. In the not too distant past, some physicians and other health care professionals thought that the less patients knew about their condition, the better would be their chances of recovery. Some health care professionals would even withhold information of impending death, fearing that such knowledge might lead a person to despair. Because of an awakened moral sense on the part of health care professionals and a sharper realization that patients have legal and moral rights that must be respected, there is now a much greater tendency to be open and honest concerning patients' conditions, the purpose of the proposed treatment, and the treatment prognosis. *The Patient's Bill of Rights* of the American Hospital Association states:

> The patient has the right to obtain
> from the physician complete current
> information concerning diagnosis,
> treatment, and prognosis in terms the
> patient can be reasonably expected
> to understand.[1]

Principles

Clearly, information on serious sickness or impending death must be furnished even if the individual does not ask for it. Legal precedent as well as moral concern prompts this realization. Hence, physicians and other health care professionals may not defend their lack of communication by pleading that the patient did not wish to know and did not ask questions. In some hospitals, a patients' representative helps patients understand their situation, especially when surgery is anticipated. Whenever possible, the leader of the health care team, the physician, should be involved in explaining the situation to the patient.

Although health care professionals usually respect

patients' rights insofar as providing the proper information, difficult situations often arise and health care professionals hesitate to tell patients their true condition. For example, patients with serious cases of cancer might become despondent and even suicidal if they know their true situation. With this in mind, *The Patient's Bill of Rights* states:

> When it is not medically advisable to give such information to the patient, the information should be made available to an appropriate person in his or her behalf.[2]

Discussion

Although well-intentioned, this statement is unsatisfactory and incomplete. It seems to indicate that when health care professionals feel that harm might result if the patient knows the truth, they fulfill their obligation by telling some friend or family member about the patient's condition and prognosis. The statement does not indicate, however, what the family member or the friend is supposed to do once the information has been communicated. In order to ensure proper respect for the patient, another dimension of the situation must be explored.

Even though the medical personnel might fear untoward results if patients are informed of their true condition, it does not mean that patients should never be told the truth. Indeed, health care professionals should remember in these cases the words of Eric Cassell, MD:

> The depression in patients that commonly occurs after the diagnosis of a fatal disease seems to stem in part from the conspiracy of silence. The physician can be a great help by simply making it clear to the patient that he is available for open and direct communication.[3]

Interviews with ill or dying patients reveal that they do not wish to be kept continually in doubt about their condition; on the other hand, they do not want it revealed to them in an abrupt or brutal manner. According to Howard Brody, MD:

> A decision to reveal a grave prognosis, which may be "ethical" in itself, may become "unethical" if the physician tells the patient bluntly and then withdraws, without offering any emotional support to help the patient resolve his feelings. In fact, the assurance that the physician plans to see it through along with the patient, and that he will always make himself available to offer any comfort possible, may be more important than the bad news itself. In many of the "sour cases" that are offered as justification for withholding the truth, it may well be the absence of this transmission of compassion, rather than the telling of the truth, that produced the unfortunate result.[4]

Because physicians are not always able to convey information concerning serious illness or impending death in a fitting manner, a person trained in the dynamics of accepting sickness and death is useful in the present-day hospital setting. Crisis counseling of this nature is not an arcane art, but, on the other hand, one must be prepared competently in order to perform it well. Well-meaning but untrained people can do more harm than good when trying to help in crises.

Conclusion

In summary, it is clear that because of the general public's increased knowledge of psychology and greater regard for the subjective process that accompanies sickness and dying, the ethical question in regard to truth telling has changed. The question should not be "Should we tell?" but rather, "How do we share this information with the patient?"

1. "The Patient's Bill of Rights," American Hospital Association, 1973.
2. "Patient's Bill of Rights."
3. Eric Cassell, *The Healer's Art* (Philadelphia: J. B. Lippincott, 1976), p. 197.
4. Howard Brody, *Ethical Decisions in Medicine* (Boston: Little, Brown & Co., 1976), p. 40.

Confidentiality 16

From the Hippocratic oath to modern ethical codes, confidentiality has been a concern. The fundamental aim of confidentiality is to foster communication of important, sometimes intimate, information which will help a professional aid a client or patient. Confidentiality is a concern for lawyers, teachers, and other professionals. Because the medical relationship is especially sensitive, confidentiality in regard to patients' diagnosis and prognosis is an important value. Thus, confidentiality, in an effort to foster trust, excludes unauthorized persons from gaining access to patient information and requires that people who have such information legitimately refrain from communicating it to others.

Numerous examples of the difficulty of protecting confidential information have surfaced. Recently a technician leaked information about a possible bone marrow donor in California to a young man dying of leukemia in Texas. Court battles were waged for two months because of this breach of confidential records stored in a university computer bank. Does a minor have the right to physician consultation and confidentiality without parental involvement where birth control devices are desired? What are the rights of psychiatric patients in relationship to their files? Can third party payers of medical care demand a copy of the patient's medical records before payment is made? In modern technological medicine, how many people actually have access to a patient's records? Siegler, in 1982, related that one patient who underwent an elective cholecystectomy complained about the number of people writing in or examining his chart. A survey estimated that at least seventy-five people need access to provide quality care.[1] Are the above examples indications that confidentiality can no longer be guaranteed and is therefore a defunct ethical requirement in the medical profession?

Principles

Confidentiality in the medical transaction can be crucial to the goals of the physician and the patient. If the patient does not believe that the physician will maintain confidences, he or she may not supply possibly embarrassing or personal information important for good history taking and diagnostic procedures. Likewise, confidentiality is important during the treatment period, since physician-patient interactions depend on trust. This crucial element of trust in the physician-patient relationship could be damaged in the overall concern for a patient's health. A number of relationships are at stake if trust is broken: patient-physician, patient and all other health care providers, the reputation of the physician in the community, and his or her relationship with other patients. Ultimately privacy, personal autonomy, the decision-making process for physician and patient, the patient's responsibility for his or her own health, and public health values could be threatened.

Discussion

Very often, many people need access to medical records in order to ensure proper care for patients. In health care facilities where there is a team of healers, all must have access to needed information. Groups of subspecialists, attending physicians, medical students, three shifts of nurses, and a variety of auxiliary services—each necessary to care for a patient—must have access to records that chart the patient's progress. Simplistic solutions to the issue of confidentiality should be avoided. It would be dangerous to isolate information into different compartments as if the patient were not a whole person or as if one could cure the person by attending only to the physical or the social or the psychological dimensions of the patient's life. Although many providers may be involved in care, this does not mean that idle curiosity or simple interest is sufficient reason to have access to a patient's chart. This must be kept in mind by the administrative auditors who have some need to examine a chart and by the health care professionals on the floor who are caring for the patient. Better health care through a number of specialists, especially in a university setting, must balance carefully the patient's right to confidentiality and the need for information.

Computerization of medical records also increases the potential for breaches of confidentiality. Although the latest technology may make the storing and retrieving of valuable information more efficient and less cumbersome, the director of medical records must provide a network to protect privacy. Physicians may usually depend on this when they are in an institutional setting, but they should remember that in private practice it is their responsibility to ensure the safety of this information. This may be difficult when a central computer bank is used, especially when not all the users are physicians.

Another issue, which is more controllable, is the self-discipline required by all when dealing with patient information. Where something is said—in the cafeteria, in the hall, in the elevator—can be crucial. It is not ethical to allow indiscriminate conversation to take place in and out of health care facilities that violates any patient's right to confidentiality. This is pertinent with cases used in classrooms, rounds, literature, and other teaching areas. One should be careful to mask the identity of those whose cases are used in order to respect their right to confidentiality.

Confidentiality has its limits. Increased access is the result of modern medicine, as seen above, because quality care is ensured only through a larger number of people having access to a patient's chart. Without greater access, care could be compromised. There are classic cases as well. When the patient threatens suicide, for example, confidentiality must be broken to prevent harm to the patient and to other members of society. Such a threat may even be an indirect plea for help. Physicians must be careful to avoid allowing personal biases to interfere with patient decision making in "allowing to die" situations, which may seem to be suicide but are not. Similarly, public health laws require a breaking of confidentiality to prevent harm to society or to innocent third parties. Such is the case with suspected child abuse, contagious disease, or persons that threaten the life of other members of society.

Conclusion

Confidentiality is meant to protect persons and the relationships that they have with health care providers to ensure trust and patient autonomy and to provide security as health care is given. Modern technological medicine poses a new challenge to older concepts of confidentiality narrowly inscribed in the one-on-one model of health care. Nonetheless, the values that confidentiality was supposed to foster still exist, and their protection must be reexamined in contemporary settings so that the patient's health may continue to be served.

1. Mark Siegler, "Confidentiality in Medicine—A Decrepit Concept," *New England Journal of Medicine* 309(1982): 1518-1521.

Allowing a Person to Die 17

One serious problem in medical ethics arises in many different settings. In the neonatal nursery, the oncology ward, the surgical intensive care unit, a long term care facility, or a private home, health care professionals often must decide when to allow a person to die.

Principles

When is it moral or ethical to stop prolonging life and allow a person, whether old or young, to die? This is allowable in two situations: (1) when the treatment to prolong life would be useless; and, (2) when prolonging life would cause a serious burden for the patient. Useless treatment is any treatment that does not benefit the patient as a person. For example, a patient near death from kidney failure need not be treated with antibiotics if he contracts pneumonia, because there is no surety that such treatment would prolong life for any significant time. Moreover, when death is imminent and the patient is clearly in an irreversible coma, aggressive efforts to prolong life would be useless because longer life would not benefit the patient.

Determining when medical treatment or therapy would be a serious burden to a patient is a different matter. When we judge a treatment to be useless, we assume that death is imminent and that the treatment will not prolong life for any significant time. But there are many situations in which life could be prolonged through medical treatment but either the treatment or the results of the treatment might cause a serious burden for the patient. Consider, for example, a patient with brain cancer: surgery to remove the growth is possible, but, even if successful, there is a possibility of partial paralysis and blindness. One may refuse such life-prolonging treatment because of the serious burden that might result. The decisive factor here is not the benefit of prolonged life that might result from the surgery, but the burden the treatment itself might impose on the person. Such a refusal of treatment is not the equivalent of suicide. On the contrary, it should be considered as an acceptance of the human condition, or a wish to avoid the application of a procedure disproportionate to the results that can be expected. Even the desire not to impose excessive expense on the family or the community may be a legitimate reason for refusing life-prolonging care because the compassionate person includes the needs and rights of others when making an ethical decision.

Discussion

In order to determine in an ethical and compassionate manner whether treatment is useless or involves a grave burden, the following considerations may be helpful:

1. The reason we can judge ethically that prolonging life is useless or would involve a serious burden is because human life is not the ultimate good, nor the greatest value. Merely maintaining life, especially at the biological level, is not the purpose of human life. Life, health, and all temporal goods are subordinated to the purpose of life. People may differ in defining the purpose of life: some may define it as sapient life, others as the potential for interpersonal relationships, and others as spiritual growth and development. But all seem to agree that when the purpose of life cannot be achieved, then the duty to prolong life is no longer present.

2. The basis for the patient-physician relationship is a promise by the physician to do what is best for the patient. Usually this means that the physician and other members of the health care team try to promote physiological function and prolong life. Indeed, this is the specific purpose of the health care profession. Only in exceptional cases, then, will the decision to allow a person to die be ethically justified. This decision must be made carefully and for each person. Thus no class of people, with certain specified symptoms, can be classified *a priori* as not suitable for life-prolonging care.

3. In such an important decision, the patient should not only be consulted but given the right to make the final decision. This right also follows from the nature of the patient-physician relationship. Often, however, the person about whom the decision must be made is not conscious, either because of

temporary or permanent brain damage or undeveloped psychic capacity. In these cases, the patient's family, with the advice of the medical and pastoral team, has the right to make the final decision, provided family members are seeking the good of the patient. In forming this decision, family members should include financial concerns and other important factors that a prudent person would consider, but they must be careful not to put their self-interest before that of the patient. If medical personnel believe firmly that the patient's rights are being violated, they should express their concern, even through an appeal to civil authority.

4. There is a great difference between allowing a person to die and putting a person to death. One who understands this distinction would not allow an otherwise healthy person to die simply because the person could not feed himself or herself. Determining that a retarded child with duodenal atresia should starve to death, for example, is not a justifiable decision. The surgery to correct the atresia and thus prolong life should be performed because it cannot be shown that such treatment is useless nor that life for a retarded person is a serious burden.

5. If doubt exists whether the treatment would be useless or would cause a serious burden, the patient should be given the benefit of the doubt and life should be prolonged. Often the uncertainty will result from the lack of a clear medical diagnosis or prognosis. Those who work with the newborn offer many examples of newborns with a doubtful life expectancy who, after receiving aggressive care, made stunning progress.

6. Even though aggressive efforts to prolong life may be foregone because they would either be useless or involve a serious burden, the care that will mitigate suffering must be offered. Hence, patients should be bathed and given food, water, and medication, even if such medication might indirectly shorten life.

Conclusion

Allowing oneself or another to die is a very serious ethical decision. The foregoing principles, based on the purpose of human life and the physician-patient relationship, will not make such decisions easy; however, they do offer direction toward solutions that enable the health care professional to be aware that he or she is striving for what is best for the patient.

Ordinary and Extraordinary Means 18

When discussing the care of a dying patient, people often use the terms *ordinary* and *extraordinary* means as though they solve all ethical questions. But closer analysis often reveals that the terms do not lead to a clear solution. Are the terms useful or meaningful in ethical discourse? They seem to be, if a few distinctions are kept in mind.

Principles

Clearly, physicians and ethicists approach the dying patient with different emphases; the ethicist is more concerned with how the person dies, and the physician is more concerned with how to prolong life. When particular ethical cases are being decided, it seems that there need not be any radical disagreement between physicians and ethicists if three truths are clearly distinguished:

1. Physicians and moralists often use the terms *ordinary means* and *extraordinary means* with different connotations.

2. Although the physician has the expertise and the right to make decisions concerning the usefulness of medical effects of some particular means, the patient (or the patient's family) has the right to determine whether a particular means is ordinary or extraordinary from an ethical point of view.

3. If the means are determined from an ethical point of view to be ordinary, then they must be employed; if determined to be extraordinary, they may or may not be employed, the decision being made by the patient (or the family) in consultation with the physician, but ordinary care should continue.

Discussion

In order to explain these distinctions more clearly, the following thoughts are offered.

Physicians often use the term *ordinary means* to describe an accepted or standard medical procedure. A procedure that is new and untested, still in the experimental stage, is called *extraordinary* or heroic. Thus from the physician's point of view, most means could be classified as ordinary or extraordinary without any reference to the patient. From a medical perspective, then, a respirator, tube feeding, or use of an artificial heart have at one time been extraordinary but became ordinary by reason of effectiveness and acceptability.

The ethicist, on the other hand, sees these terms in a different light. For the ethicist, ordinary and extraordinary means have no meaning unless the patient's condition is known. For example, one cannot denominate a respirator or tube feeding ordinary or extraordinary from an ethical perspective unless the patient's diagnosis and prognosis is known. The ethicist assumes that a person has a need or obligation to prolong human life, but that there are limits to this need or obligation (see p. 66). One obvious limit is that one need not do something useless to prolong life. Thus, if a patient dying of cancer contracts pneumonia, it is generally agreed that one may refuse treatment for pneumonia if life would not be prolonged for a significant time. Hence one need not seek all possible cures for a fatal condition if there is little hope that any of them would be successful.

Another limit to the obligation of prolonging life occurs when the means to prolong life would involve a grave burden to the person insofar as striving for the more important values of life are concerned. For example, classical ethicists maintained that a surgical procedure might be declared extraordinary because of the concomitant burden it might involve. Today we might declare a quadruple amputation extraordinary from an ethical perspective not because of the actual pain of the surgery, but because of the burden that life in this condition might impose on the person.

In maintaining that one is free to make a judgment not to prolong life because a grave burden would result, even though prolonging life is possible, we are affirming that, although human life is a great good, it is not the greatest good. This is the practical meaning of the word *burden*: making it difficult for one to attain the purpose of life.

Ethically speaking, then, ordinary means of preserving life are the medicines, treatments, and operations that offer a reasonable hope of benefit for the patient or that can be obtained or used without excessive expense, pain, or burden. Extraordinary means are the medicines, treatments, and operations that cannot be used or obtained without excessive expense, pain, or other burden or that do not offer a reasonable hope of benefit.

Some ethicists maintain that the terms ordinary and extraordinary are inadequate for the decision-making task in ethics. It seems the theoretical difficulties could be eliminated if the first question is not: Is this means ordinary or extraordinary? but, rather: Is there an obligation to prolong life? Thus the patient's condition and value system must first be discerned. If the answer to this latter question is affirmative, then the medical means necessary to prolong life are ordinary means from an ethical perspective. If there is no obligation to prolong life, then only procedures that will keep the patient comfortable are ordinary means and all other means are extraordinary from an ethical perspective.

The practical difficulties in applying the distinction between ordinary and extraordinary means to prolong life will always remain. Determining whether it is time to allow oneself to die, or to allow another to die, will always be a complex decision for a compassionate person. This is especially true if the decision involves discontinuing a means already in use. This difficulty is evidenced excruciatingly in the case of newborns with birth defects. The difficulties do not destroy the use of the distinction, however.

Clearly, the physician is responsible for deciding which therapies are ordinary and which are extraordinary, but who is responsible for deciding this matter from the ethical perspective? The physician must be involved in the decision because the diagnosis and prognosis will depend mainly upon his or her science and skill, but the patient has the ultimate responsibility for making this decision. The patient retains this responsibility not only because he or she has the right to determine which values will be pursued, but because only the patient knows the other circumstances, for example, the pain, expense, or inconvenience involved in a particular therapy, which must be considered in making the ethical decision.

More difficult problems arise when the patient is incompetent and cannot make the ethical decision. Some would refer all the decisions to the courts, but it seems the courts should be consulted only when a manifest injustice might be inflicted on an incompetent patient. More often, the family or spouse should decide for the incompetent patient for two reasons: (1) they love the patient and will decide what is best for the person; and (2) they know the patient's mind and should be able to request what he or she would want. Physicians and family members should cooperate in the decision-making process, with neither group asserting an adversarial position, but with both groups seeking to make decisions beneficial for the patient.

The Quality of Life 19

The terms *quality of life* and *sanctity of life* are used as a rallying point for opposite opinions in questions that arise at the beginning and end of life. Careful analysis of the concepts and the underlying issues of dealing with dying patients may help clarify some of the ambiguity of this debate.

Principles

The term *sanctity of life* usually has been interpreted to mean that each individual, regardless of the state of health, is valuable, is not to be used as a means, and is to be treated with dignity. This value depends on the transcendence of God, an inner spiritual center, or the dynamic of personality that transcends each person. With this concept, the refusal or withdrawal of medical care based solely on the individual's lack of ability to realize full human potential is morally unacceptable. Difficulties arise, however, when the term is taken to an extreme. Those who say that because of the sanctity of life no treatment should ever be stopped or withheld, for example, in the case of a dying patient or defective newborn, advocate vitalism. This position preserves physical existence, even when other goods in life cannot or can no longer be realized. According to this position, the mere prolongation of physical life is morally required without asking pertinent questions about the goals and purposes of life. This position prevents good medical decision making.

The term *quality of life* usually has been interpreted to mean that the value of an individual's life is determined in part by that individual's ability to realize certain goals in life. When these abilities no longer exist or cannot exist, then the obligations to prolong life or to continue treatment do not exist. In the extreme, this concept can establish arbitrary and unjust criteria in medical decision making, for instance, that all mentally disabled individuals or all individuals suffering from certain genetic defects should not receive medical treatment. In addition, this concept usually states that this decision or judgment is in the patient's best interest; however, confusion often surrounds whose "best interest" is really at stake.

Additional implications of these terms are often confusing. Quality of life versus sanctity of life arguments mean that one chooses quality rather than quantity; that one does not respect life and the other does; that one is not consistent about value judgments while the other is. Each of these distinctions is a false dichotomy.

Discussion

The question raised in either the quality or sanctity of life concept is a question concerning the morally significant in determining whether to treat aggressively, withhold, or withdraw certain therapies. At issue is the relationship between biological life and other human qualities and the significance that this relationship has in the medical decision-making process. Some distinctions may make this point clear.

First, one should be clear about the descriptive and normative ways in which the concepts are employed. Both can be used in a descriptive fashion, as in the following two sentences: The life of the paraplegic is sacred and should be treated with dignity. The paraplegic's quality of life may be different from someone who does not share the same impairment. Both statements are descriptive. Neither tells a practitioner exactly what to do; they are not normative. This descriptive function is important if one is to make a good and ethical medical judgment. Confusion arises when one interprets this descriptive function into an ethical imperative, such as do or do not treat or treat aggressively, without asking other questions.

Second, the purpose of medical care is patient benefit. The reason for treating a patient is to free the patient from the types of impairments that prevent other important values from being realized. Medicine works to eradicate these impairments to full life for the patient's benefit, but in working to eliminate impairments, medicine cannot choose to eliminate the individuals who have these impairments. Such actions are contrary to medicine itself. Also, one must remember that dying is the last act of living. Unnecessary death can be averted, but death is an inevitable reality for us all. Helping people to die well, whether they are young or old, is a vital part of medicine. When these factors are considered carefully, one realizes that the "quality" of a person's life is at the center of medical practice. Benefitting a person medically means aiding the person to realize the qualities or goals of biological existence and not solely to prolong physiological existence.

Third, decision making in difficult circumstances is a crucial part of medical practice. Medical care is an art, a science, and a process of making sound decisions with a patient toward the realization of important life goals. The patient's ability to realize certain goals in life is significant. The dying cancer patient, for example, may be allowed to die because no effective cures or treatments are available and because continued treatment merely prolongs the dying process. The pain and the "quality" of the person's life due to this illness does not justify prolonging mere physical existence. Respect for the sacredness and dignity of the person requires allowing the patient to die, withholding certain therapies, or withdrawing some because they do not promote life. Aggressive treatment in such a case is unethical.

Conclusion

The quality of a person's life is not synonymous with full physiological, psychological, or emotional life. One is respected as a person regardless of the degree to which one attains such functions; however, the degree to which one realizes these functions plays a significant role in the medical decision-making process. To neglect completely such factors is to be a vitalist, using the technologies of medicine as a mechanic rather than as a physician. The central focus of medical decisions is the benefit of the patient, which includes the patient's ability to pursue the goals of life. The quality of the patient's life as it relates to realizing life's goals is central to sound ethical-medical decision making. Quality and sanctity of life are not opposites; they only become so in oversimplified arguments. What is crucial is that good decision making occur based on basic principles of justice. Perhaps it is not quality and sacredness that cause conflict in these decisions, but a lack of reason and justice.

Human Experimentation 20

When science takes man as its
subject, tensions arise between two
values basic to Western Society:
freedom of scientific inquiry and
protection of individuals' inviolability.[1]

That research on human beings is often useful and
necessary for the common good is undeniable. Many
beneficial vaccines and other therapies, such as smallpox and
poliomyelitis vaccines, open heart surgery, and successful
treatment of certain birth defects, have required human
research and the whole world attests to its value. But there is
no doubt that occasionally human research has been abused.
The world will never forget the horrors of the human research
inflicted on innocent human beings in the name of scientific
progress in the Nazi concentration camps. Aside from such
atrocities, other egregious violations of human rights have
occurred in the United States, such as the withholding of newly
discovered penicillin from patients in the Tuskeegee syphillis
study, the Willowbrook experiments in which retarded children
were used as experimental subjects, and the injection of live
cancer cells in unknowing subjects in the Jewish Chronic
Disease Hospital case.[2]

Psychological research has also given rise to serious
debate about behavior control of debilitated patients. Abuses
arising from human research are not usually the product of
demented or perverted minds; rather they result from lack of
care and ethical sensitivity on the part of researchers who
overlook the rights of human beings in an effort to ensure
scientific progress or enhance personal prestige.[3]

Research on human subjects should be clearly
distinguished from therapy for human subjects since the
primary purpose of research is not to heal but to learn. Yet it is
helpful and valid from an ethical perspective to classify human
research as either *therapeutic* or *nontherapeutic*. One may
assume greater risks if the research is directed toward healing
as well as knowledge. Thus, therapeutic research studies the
effects of using diagnostic, prophylactic, or therapeutic
methods that depart from standard medical practice but hold

out a reasonable expectation of success. Clearly, what begins as human therapeutic research may later become standard medical treatment. Nontherapeutic research, on the other hand, is not designed to improve the health of the research subjects. Rather it seeks to gain knowledge or develop techniques that may benefit people other than the subjects of the research project.

Principles

The proper manner of conducting research on various categories of human subjects has become one of the most discussed bioethical questions of recent years. Through international seminars and studies on the subject, some ethical principles have been developed to serve as a guide for researchers and for those who support research. In all, we list eight ethical norms for research which involves human subjects.

Norm 1. The knowledge sought through research must be important and not obtainable by other means, and the research must be carried on by qualified people.

Norm 2. Appropriate experimentation upon animals and cadavers must precede human experimentation.

Norm 3. The risk of suffering or injury must be proportionate to the good to be gained. This norm is significant for conducting nontherapeutic and therapeutic research.

Norm 4. Subjects should be selected so that risks and benefits will not fall unequally upon one group in society. Hence the poor and weak and disabled should not be disproportionately enlisted as subjects of research.

Norm 5. In order to protect the integrity of the human person, free and informed (voluntary) consent must be obtained. Proxy consent must be obtained if subjects cannot give informed consent.

Norm 6. At any time during the course of research, the subject (or the guardian who has given proxy consent) must be free to terminate the subject's participation in the experiment.

Norm 7. In psychological research, the researcher must work *with* not *on* the human subject.

Norm 8. The researcher must avoid breaking down human trust by lying or manipulation. However, subjects can give free and informed consent to experiments in which they may be given ambiguous communication if they are warned beforehand.

Discussion

Some special problems of research should be mentioned. Because discussion of the relationship between risk and potential benefit is most important for discerning the limits of human research, the possible ill effects of the research must be delineated beforehand as clearly as possible. Sometimes, as in the case of the poliomyelitis inoculation in 1954 when the use of some poorly prepared live vaccine resulted in the death of children or in the case of the 1980 Swine Flu inoculation disaster, the risks are far greater than predicted. Hence, absolute certainty in regard to the nature and degree of the risk cannot be required. To demand such certitude would paralyze all scientific research and would very often be detrimental to the patient. Care must be taken, however, to predict as accurately as possible the nature and magnitude of risk from any particular human experiment and to reveal it completely to the subjects. When discussing risk, it is important to distinguish between the frequency of a risk and the gravity of a risk. Thus, a researcher may state that a risk is "light" if it happens in only three or four percent of cases. But if the risk in question is death or serious impairment, then it is a grave risk and may not be justified by reason of the benefit.

When determining the degree of risk that a person might undergo, one must always bear in mind the difference between therapeutic and nontherapeutic research. If the research project is therapeutic, then persons may undergo greater risk because one is seeking to avoid personal impairment or death through participating in the research projects.

Another ethical issue arises due to double-blind research. The objectivity of scientific research depends largely upon the use of controlled experimentation in which a group of experimental subjects is divided into two subgroups, one of which receives the experimental therapy while the other, the control group, receives the standard therapy or a placebo. This sometimes is called a randomized clinical trial. Sometimes double-blind control is used; thus not only are subjects not informed as to which kind of treatment they have received, but also even those researchers who evaluate the effects of the treatments do not know which subjects have received which treatment. Only the double-blind technique can eliminate the placebo effect, that is, the improvement frequently experienced by patients who expect it and the effect of bias on the part of the researchers. Double-blind procedures raise ethical questions, however, since it would seem (1) that those patients who do not receive the new therapy are at a therapeutic disadvantage; and (2) that none of the participants in the double-blind experiment could have given informed consent to a specific treatment.

Hence, in double-blind experiments the subjects should be informed that if they consent to the experiment some will receive the new treatment and others will not, but that none of the subjects will know. The potential subjects will then be free to consent to these experimental conditions or to refuse to participate. If the clinical trial involves a placebo for the control group, and the project aims at finding an agent that will mitigate or cure a lethal or disabling disease, then a special ethical issue arises. Most likely, the control groups will not be involved in a therapeutic program because they are not receiving a valid therapy for their illness or disease. This is especially true if there is some justification for thinking that the new therapy might be effective. Thus the same protocol may be therapeutic for some and nontherapeutic for others. For this reason researchers then must be doubly cautious when a double-blind placebo protocol is being designed or reviewed. If the new therapy proves effective, then the program should be discontinued and all subjects should be given the new and effective therapy. Rash decisions as to what constitutes effective therapy, however, should be avoided.

Puzzling problems in research also occur when one person gives consent for an incompetent person for whom the first person is morally responsible. Thus a parent gives consent for an infant or child and a husband or wife for a comatose spouse. Such consent is commonly called *proxy consent*. Decisions of proxy consent must be made in view of the good of the individual incompetent person, not for society's good, for a class good, nor for the good of the person who acts as proxy. Otherwise the incompetent person is manipulated and treated as a thing. If the research is therapeutic there would be reason for the proxy to allow risk in proportion to the good that might accrue to the incompetent individual. If the research is nontherapeutic, however, then the decision is more difficult.

Conclusion

In order to obviate excesses in research and to facilitate scientific progress, the federal government monitors research protocols through the Federal Drug Administration (FDA) and by requiring that each research institution have an Institutional Review Board (IRB) to evaluate research protocols. For the most part, the FDA is concerned with approving new drugs and devices and the IRBs seek to ensure that the human subjects give free and informed consent, that the risks are justified by potential benefits, and that the research protocol will achieve its stated purpose.

1. Jay Katz, *Experimentation with Human Beings*, (New York: Sage Foundation, 1972), p. 1.
2. Katz.
3. M. F. Shapiro and R. P. Charnow, "Scientific Misconduct in Investigational Drug Trials," *New England Journal of Medicine*, 312(1985): 731-736.

At times people are reluctant to release the body of a loved one for autopsy. Are there good reasons for this reluctance? Is it a violation of propriety, ethics, or religion to release the body of a spouse, parent, or child for medical examination? If not, why the continued reluctance?

Principles

When a human being dies, the body is no longer unified by the lifegiving principle or soul by which it is a constituted human being. The cadaver of a person, then, is not a *human* body in the proper sense of the word. Insofar as possible, we should avoid referring to the physical remains of a person as though the person existed *in* a human body or was, so to speak, limited by the human body. Although existing in this life, the human person is a substantial unity of spirit (form) and body (matter), not an accidental juxtaposition of two distinct entities.[1] Although the remains of a human body may resemble the body of a living person, and although this resemblance may be prolonged through embalming, the remains are not a *human* body, but a mass of organic matter, decomposing into constitutive organic elements.

If the corpse of a human person is not a human body, why are people so concerned about proper care for the remains of the deceased person? Why treat it with the respect and reverence that it usually receives? Respect and reverence are due the remains of a human being because of the value of human life that once informed the now inert mass still bearing the image of the deceased person. In order to mourn and express sorrow for the fact that the person will no longer be present in the same manner as before, certain reverential actions are performed that express the love of the people who remain. Respect for the dead body, then, signifies respect for human life, respect for God, and respect for the person who once subsisted with this now corrupting corpse and who now exists in a different modality. Hence the actions, the ritual that people follow when caring for the body of a deceased person, have a meaning beyond their apparent signification.

Autopsy is the examination of a cadaver after death performed in order to provide greater medical knowledge concerning the cause of death. Historically, the first major impetus for autopsies was provided when Frederick II, emperor of the Holy Roman Empire, instructed physicians studying at Salerno and Naples to spend at least one year in the study of anatomy. Theologians expressed the belief that such dissection of the human cadaver could be done with proper respect for the dead as long as the organs were restored to the body before burial.

In accord with the respect due the remains of a human being, then, in an autopsy no organ should be removed from a corpse nor should the body be dismembered in any way unless there is a sufficient reason to justify such an action. Usually the next of kin or the person to whom the corpse is committed for care has the legal right to determine if organs may be removed from the body and if an autopsy may be performed (*Pierce v. Swan Point, 1872*). The right of the next of kin in regard to caring for the human body is not absolute, however. It may be superseded by statements made by the person while still alive, such as a wish to donate his or her body for scientific study, or by the needs of society, such as when an autopsy might help improve medical knowledge.

Today, the benefit of an autopsy occasionally will be to provide knowledge about a rare or contagious disease. In such cases autopsies should be performed because the good of the community demands it and because increased medical knowledge is needed. If the next of kin were not willing to approve the autopsy, the court could order that the autopsy be performed. In cases of violent death or unattended death an autopsy is required by law, no matter what wishes are expressed by the next of kin.

Usually, however, the purpose of an autopsy is not to trace the etiology of a rare disease or to discover unknown or violent causes of death. More frequently, autopsies are performed to help health care professionals achieve a higher level of effectiveness in the care of the living. Autopsies are especially useful for the common good when performed in teaching hospitals. The autopsy rate of a hospital is usually a sign of concern for excellence and offers a gauge of professional integrity and interest in scientific advancement. Through autopsies, the diagnosis and treatment a person received can be evaluated and staff members encouraged to observe a high level of proficiency.

Discussion

From a Christian point of view, the practice of allowing autopsies on one's body for scientific research is acceptable and even to be encouraged if a true need exists. Pope Pius XII, for example, exhibited approval of autopsies when he said:

> The public must be educated. It must be explained with intelligence and respect that to consent explicitly or tacitly to serious damage to the integrity of the corpse in the interest of those who are suffering, is no violation of the reverence due to the dead.[2]

According to the prevailing opinion of Jewish scholars, autopsies can be condoned only when there are indications that the information accruing from them may be of value in saving the life of another individual. Thus postmortem dissections are indicated when an experimental drug or surgical procedure was used and the autopsy is likely to shed some light on the merits of the treatment. Similarly, when death was caused by contagious disease or genetic disorder, autopsies are warranted for the purpose of instituting prophylactic treatment or helping with genetic counseling. Most rabbinic authorities also permit postmortem dissection for forensic purposes when mandated by law. In all cases where autopsies are indicated, they must be limited to the special areas where relevant information may be obtained. After the examination, all organs must be returned for burial.[3]

The teaching of Islam does not allow for voluntary autopsy because it is considered a desecration of the human person who was associated with the body. If the law requires it, however, then the next of kin may acquiesce to it. Unless some law would be broken or public health endangered, it seems the religious beliefs of people who disapprove of autopsies should be respected. It is worthwhile to point out, however, that one reason why medicine in the Islamic world failed to progress after a promising beginning was due to a lack of clinical information that could have been garnered through autopsies.[4]

Because of what it represents, a corpse should be shown respect and reverence. Such respect and reverence is consistent with autopsies that are designed to promote public health and improve medical knowledge, provided proper respect is shown for the cadavers. When people are faced with a decision concerning autopsy, they should be encouraged to approve such a procedure because of the help that will be offered to others.

1. E. Cassell, "The Nature of Suffering and the Goals of Medicine," *New England Journal of Medicine* 306 (1981): 639-645.
2. Pope Pius XII, *The Human Body* (Boston: St. Paul Press, 1960): p. 382.
3. "Cadavers," *Encyclopedia of Bioethics, vol. I*; p. 144.
4. "Islam," *Encyclopedia of Bioethics, vol. II*; p. 788.

Counseling and Values 22

In our pluralistic society, health care professionals are often called on to counsel or advise people who have a value system different than their own. Patients or clients seek help in making difficult decisions with ethical implications, such as, whether to have children, seek a divorce, have potentially debilitating surgery, allow an infant or an aged parent to die, or have an abortion. What is the health care professional's ethical responsibility when this conflict of value systems occurs? Can the responsible person say, "I leave my values at home when I put on my white coat"? This approach is insufficient because it leads to a form of schizophrenia, forcing a person to stifle conscience when carrying out one's professional responsibilities. Moreover, it implies that there is such a thing as a value-free profession. What, then, should the ethical health care professional do in the face of value conflict? Declare from the beginning where he or she stands on a particular point, and then invite the patient to state his case? Obviously not, because this attitude would hamper the relationship that a counselor must foster in order to help a person make decisions. In order to present a more workable method, we shall review a few principles of counseling.

Principles

Two fundamental types of counseling exist: spiritual counseling and ethical counseling. Spiritual counseling is concerned with instilling, strengthening, or changing values. A spiritual counselor, sometimes called a spiritual director, is concerned with instructing people in regard to the goals of life and with increasing their affection for these goals. In order to increase commitment to goals, he or she will instruct people but also dispose the person seeking help to appreciate and experience the goodness, beauty, and effectiveness of the goals in question. In addition, spiritual counseling focuses on the rewards, whether transcendent or temporal, that result from dedication to a particular value system.

Ethical counseling is concerned with helping people make informed and free decisions in accord with their own personal value systems. The ethical counselor presupposes that the other person has a valid value system, and the counselor's task is to help the person judge and act in accord with that system if at all possible. With this in mind, the ethical counselor has a threefold function:

1. Offering knowledge necessary for ethical questions (e.g., what will a possible surgery involve);
2. Helping the counselee understand the options available and the predicted results of these actions (e.g., what methods of family limitation are available and what are the physical and psychological results); and
3. Helping the client make free decisions; that is, decisions free of family, peer, or emotional pressure or compulsion (e.g., helping a family realize that only unconscious guilt feelings keep them from removing useless life-support systems).

This last function is the most important and most difficult of the three. It involves the essence of ethical counseling — to help free another from emotional conflict, confusion, or unconscious fear or guilt that so often accompanies a significant ethical decision. The result of ethical counseling may be a decision accompanied by emotion, but the decision should not be dominated by emotion or unconscious drives.

Discussion

Do health care professionals act as spiritual or ethical counselors? Usually they act as ethical counselors, but a patient will sometimes approach a health care professional asking the type of direction or advice that indicates a desire for spiritual counseling. The health care professional must determine which type of counseling is involved by reason of the situation and the type of questions asked. Some may not feel capable of counseling from a spiritual viewpoint; some may not feel capable of counseling from an ethical viewpoint. We believe that spiritual counseling is easier than ethical counseling, especially if one has internalized a traditional religious value system. Ethical counseling usually requires special training because it involves more unconscious and, at first glance, hidden factors.

In spiritual counseling, if the counselee were to propose an action that violates the common value system, it would be the counselor's responsibility to call attention to this lack of integrity. One who acts as an ethical counselor, however, does not have this responsibility. Thus the ethical counselor will not try to change a value, nor will the ethical counselor be called on to object to the counselee's actions as long as these actions are in accord with the counselee's value system. Is this a denial of the counselor's integrity? Does this result in a denial of the counselor's own value system? One of the most important values that one should stand for is to respect the conscience of other people. Conscience is the focal point of each person's worth. Religious people believe that conscience is the contact point with God, and because of relationship to God each person has equal value. People who do not consider themselves religious recognize conscience as the source of freedom and see in the capacity for freedom the characteristic that endows each person with inalienable rights. When we respect another person's conscience, we respond to a value that transcends any one value system, and we establish a basis for human community, even in the face of disagreement about other values. We also establish a means of resolving disagreements because of the bond of community.

Although an ethical counselor respects the conscience of the counselee, he or she is not called on to help the counselee carry out the proposed action. If a person determines that he or she wishes to be allowed to die by having a life-support system disconnected, and the attending physician considers this unethical, the physician should withdraw from the case rather than compromise his or her own personal value system. If a third party might be injured as a result of a decision that a patient or client makes in good conscience, the counselor has an ethical responsibility to express disagreement and point out the injustice of the action. Otherwise, the counselor's silence might aid and abet the unjust action. In some cases there is not only an ethical but also a legal responsibility to protect a third party. In most states, for example, there are laws against aiding and abetting suicide or other serious crimes.

Conclusion

The relationship between patients and health care professionals goes beyond the bonds of technology, penetrating to the very heart of what makes us human: our conscience. Building relationships that respect the conscience of each person, both patient and professional, is a task that bespeaks the transcendent worth of health care.

Mental health is a necessity in order for people to function optimally in relationship to themselves, society, and the other social groups of life. Subsequently, when someone suffers from any mental health problem, appropriate treatment is seen as necessary. Many of the same values and characteristics that mark the physician-patient relationship in other areas of health care are present when one discusses mental health and psychiatric care. Because mental health is not merely physiological or organic, however, numerous assumptions about the person, appropriate social interaction, and society are implicit in any type of therapy. An awareness of these assumptions is important if proper care is to be given and if the dignity and worth of the person treated is to be respected.

Principles and Discussion

Counseling takes many forms and one must first clarify the kind of counseling one is seeking. Some people seek spiritual counseling as a method to identify important religious values in their faith life and to attempt to integrate spiritual values into their lives. One seeks spiritual counseling if there are values present in the person's life that the person is attempting to live more completely. Closely associated but distinct from spiritual counseling is ethical counseling or value counseling, where one is in search of some values and seeks out a person, someone "wise," to help one explore the area of values within his or her life. Ethical counseling requires imparting information that the individual in his or her questioning may not accept. Ethical counseling presumes that self-determination or autonomy is an important value that must be respected and that the person will be able to weigh various factors within his or her life as decisions are made.

Psychiatric forms of therapy deal with many problems and many areas of a person's life. Religious, spiritual, or ethical values may be part of the problems that a person wishes to resolve. In psychiatric treatment, however, the question arises as to whose values predominate and who has the "authority" to change a person's value orientation. There is a great deal of ambiguity in the psychiatric setting. Nonetheless, the basic ethical principles of autonomy, freedom of choice, and consensual communication are still a part of the relationship. When these principles are forgotten, the patient may surrender his or her autonomy unnecessarily, be falsely labeled, be excluded from future participation in social life, or not be treated with the dignity required for each human being. Psychiatric treatment, whether Freudian or behavioral, is built on certain assumptions about the human person and what is valuable in his or her personal and social life.

A first assumption is that the human being is an integrated individual with physiological, psychological, spiritual, social, and historical dimensions. When one facet of the human being suffers, the ability to realize one's values and goals in human life is hampered. This is easily seen in physiological illness. The issue becomes more complicated as one deals with the effects of social, spiritual, or psychological distortions. What kinds of "aberration" in these areas qualifies as "illness?" What is the difference between socially disapproved behavior and illness? How much idiosyncratic behavior in an individual does a society allow?

Most therapists have answered these questions to some extent, even if not with clear definitions. The therapist tries to "treat" or "help" the person in order for the person to realize some level of "well-being." There is a "prized" kind of behavior that psychiatric treatment is designed to aid. Often the person is cured when this prized behavior comes "naturally." Treatment can continue over a long period. The question is, who defines the new behavior as valuable?

Many of the individual therapies that rely on insight into one's unconscious or greater insight into the symbolic meanings of one's actions insist that wholeness is gained from this insight. The freedom that results from this insight to act and to choose from alternatives without the anxiety or other problematic behavior that brought one to seek help in the very beginning is valuable. Behavioral therapies seek ways to help the individual adapt more readily to the environment. People are not really choosers or shapers of much of their culture or history, but rather are persons capable of modifying their behavior in one way or another. This human capacity is the key to successful living and for behaviorists this is a valuable development. Other psychotherapeutic theories stress neither of these two views, but seek to understand the human being through his or her interrelation with society. Optimal functioning in the social setting then is the value to be attained. Whichever school one adheres to, one implicitly chooses certain overriding conceptions of the human being of what is to be perceived as valuable, what is important in life, and, therefore, what should be stressed.

The ethical discussion about these therapeutic values requires that one starts with and keeps central the person being treated. Like other patients, psychiatric patients are being treated to realize their well-being and their values, which may not fully match those of a given society or therapist. Care must be taken that in the process of promoting health, the therapist does not undermine the patient's values and his or her ability to choose. Undoubtedly the various schools of thought have their own values and insights. At times it is important for a person to understand why he or she acts in a certain way. At other times it is important to feel better about oneself and to have insight into the reasons for certain behaviors. At other times adaption and change are necessary. Other situations arise when one recognizes that the social systems in one's life are destructive or important and require some work and reflection. In no case does one part of the person include all his or her important values.

The values expressed in these various therapies may clash with the patient's values. The difficulty in some psychiatric treatments is the need to help the patient work out of his or her own value system, recognize distortion when it truly exists, and help the patient conform his or her life to the values that he or she pursues. There is a great deal of difference between this kind of psychiatric help and the ethical and spiritual help that the person may seek. In some cases the value and spiritual direction that an individual seeks is better given by someone other than the psychiatrist. Regardless of the type of counseling sought, the primary fact is still the centrality of the patient, the patient's needs and desires, and the values that the patient brings to the relationship.

Danger arises when people forget that any method of therapy is not truly "value neutral" or that one method of therapy is sufficient for the whole person. Often this is not the case. Ethical behavior in this area of health care requires that the therapist help the patient become more truly human (an integrated and whole person) within the scope of his or her values.

Although the field of psychiatry deals with a less empirical aspect of human existence than do other more physiological disciplines of medicine, the ethical principles remain the same. The psychiatrist, like any other physician, is in a service-oriented profession aimed at patient well-being and the pursual of patient values. This requires careful attention to the full meaning of informed consent, to the consensual working out of medical problems, and to respect for the patient's values and dignity. The nature of counseling precludes any assumption that those who do the counseling can be the value makers for a given patient. Finally, like all other dimensions of the medical profession, no one physician has the ability to meet the various needs of all the dimensions of the human being. It is through cooperation on a number of fronts, including nonmedical ones, that people may come to experience well-being.

Good Will Toward Some?

At Christmastime, whether for religious or secular reasons, most of us have a strong tendency to think of the less fortunate and to help them in one way or another. We expect this sentiment of "peace on earth, good will toward all" to be promoted by churches, synagogues, and other religious and charitable organizations. But today, for one reason or another, even radio stations and used car dealers collect food and clothing for those less fortunate. The theme of the season offers an occasion for considering some ethical issues that are closely related to "peace on earth, good will toward all" and the response to those issues that people might offer. The ethical issues under discussion are not those which might be called individual or family issues; rather, they are the issues that affect people at the social level, the systemic issues that dehumanize, deprive, and even destroy people on a grand scale. These are the macro as opposed to the micro ethical issues—the issues that affect whole nations or groups of people rather than a comparatively small percentage.

Principles

There can be no doubt that macro ethical issues affect large segments of the population today. The potential for nuclear war, the deprivation throughout the world of basic human rights, the serious problem of increasing population, the continual pollution of air and water, and the scarcity of food in some nations are all social problems that have serious ethical issues connected with them. There are no simple solutions to any of the above-mentioned problems, and as the experts seek to offer solutions, they are more insistent that most of these problems are interrelated, stifling somewhat our hopes for solution.

In this short essay, there is no possibility of suggesting solutions to these problems. Rather, let us consider options for responding or reacting to these issues. Because the world shortage of food has been featured in *Science* and in the *Annual Review of Nutrition*, we shall use this topic as the focal point of discussion.[1-3]

Discussion

What are the possible responses when a person realizes that hunger and starvation are the lot of many people in the world today and that predictions indicate the problem will increase drastically? Three responses appear to be possible:

1. To confine one's ethical concerns to one's own small world, thinking that the issue of world hunger is exaggerated by the media, or hoping that "someone will develop new technology" that will improve the production of food and eliminate hunger and starvation;

2. To maintain an interest in the macro issues of spaceship earth, relying on solutions that seem to have worked in the past. Thus one would support policies of governments or agencies that would encourage people to work harder to produce food, depending on the Lockian concept of self-interest and the conviction that there are enough resources in the world for ambitious people to feed themselves;

3. To work for the solution of the complex social issues by supporting approaches to the problem that call for a sharing of resources by developed countries with underdeveloped countries.[4]

This latter response is founded on a realization of the brotherhood of all human beings, a teaching contained in every one of the world's great religions. One who follows this response will support and join those people and organizations who suggest innovative and comprehensive solutions to the problems of society. For example, one might join the local chapter of Physicians for Social Responsibility, if concerned about nuclear war. If concerned about world hunger, people following this method of response will encourage the government of the United States "to offer not only food, but also capital, research support and educational opportunities" to people from underdeveloped countries.[5] This form of response implies that those with more will have to do with less so that everyone will have enough. Moreover, it presumes that the world has so changed and the ethical problems are so serious and complex that the resources of society are limited rather than unlimited and that the strictly economic solutions usually offered to solve ethical problems are simply insufficient because they do not provide sufficient motivation for equitable sharing of the world's goods.

Conclusion

Working with ethical problems at the macro level is a frustrating experience because individuals seem so helpless in the face of such devastating deprivation. Yet we know that many macro ethical issues of the past, such as the social injustice of slavery and the deprivation of political rights to women, have been solved or improved substantially. Moreover, most of the serious disease that devastated large numbers of people, such as smallpox and tuberculosis, and that have been conquered, were considered macro social problems 100 years ago. Hence today's macro social problems can be solved, even though they may seem insurmountable at first.

Although bettering social conditions is never easy, it is possible when fitting solutions are present and when people open their hearts and realize that all are equal and all share in the mutuality of human nature and in the love of God. At Christmastime, then, although we may not solve any of the world's problems, let us not sit on the sidelines of the struggle and merely lament the situation. Above all, although it will be painful and involve some generous sacrifices and some personal deprivation, let us become part of the solution by taking seriously this theme of the season: "Peace on Earth, Good Will Toward All."

1. L. Brown, "World Population Growth, Soil Erosion, and Food Scarcity," *Science*, 204(November 27, 1981): 995.2.
2. T. Barr, "The World Food Situation and Global Grain Products, *Science*, 214(December 4, 1981): 1087.
3. Samuel Stumpf, "The Moral Dimension of the World's Food Supply," *Annual Review of Nutrition*, (1981): 1-26.
4. Stumpf, p.18.
5. Barr, p. 1087.

Genetic Engineering 25

In Washington, DC, in May 1984, a federal judge postponed the release of a genetically engineered organism in a potato field. He declared that further consideration should be given to the effect of the organism by the environment. Dismay was expressed by the National Institute of Health and the scientists at Berkeley who were involved in the project. Ethical concern was expressed by others who maintained that because genetic engineering is still new and the full implications of new organisms and new therapies on human beings are not fully understood, caution must be exercised.

The most common objection voiced by those who oppose any kind of genetic engineering is that those involved in genetic manipulation are playing God: God alone has the "right" to develop new organisms; scientists should not manipulate DNA; human beings should accept what God has made and live according to the "nature" he has created.

A second objection is raised by those who claim that no assessment can be made of the good or bad consequences that will flow from the development of new life forms. Subsequently, nothing should be done lest a new organism be released that will be harmful to the human race or the ecological system and be resistant to any form of scientific intervention.

Another more moderate objection would allow the development and use of genetic technologies in drug development, such as interferon, and perhaps even in some new organisms that could not reproduce but would not allow the use of any genetic technologies on human beings. The consequences of tampering with the human being are simply too great. These issues demand a careful response from the scientific and medical communities and from society as a whole.

Principles

One important aspect of life is the ability to form a society that allows each person to realize his or her potential through a greater understanding of one's self and nature. These developments have led to a variety of technologies— some simple, some complex—that have made the world a more habitable place. Society has a responsibility to continue the quest to understand and to use this knowledge in a constructive manner. In genetics, this has led to greater discoveries about the building blocks of life. This does not exhaust the "secrets" or the "mysteries" of life, however. Those who assert that scientists are playing God assume that scientific knowledge unlocks all elements of being human. Such is not the case. To assume that an understanding of DNA, the ability to perfect the transfer of genetic material, or the development of new organisms leads to a complete understanding of human life is false.

The application of genetic knowledge to human beings has caused considerable concern. Purely molecular or atomistic approaches have been held out by some as a way of improving human beings; similar lines of argument by others claim genetic advancement as unethical. Scientists and critics too easily forget that the human being is also made up of nongenetic building blocks called love, friendship, faith, personality, and sociality. There is an ethical obligation for human beings to use their knowledge to protect and promote life. Genetic engineering may afford this possibility. It can be one part of exercising stewardship. The issue is not use or nonuse of genetic knowledge, but wise use that recognizes the limits and respects the multifaceted nature of the person.

There are limits, however. Perhaps science will be able to perform actions that alter basic concepts of human nature, for example, to create new life forms that are "very human" but have deliberately had rational functions suppressed so that they may more easily be manipulated. The use of greater knowledge to deny fundamental human abilities is unethical. The use of genetics that adversely affects one race, increases racial prejudice, or brands certain persons as lesser beings would also be unethical. Working within these limits should not be confused with "playing God."

Discussion

Measuring consequences of genetic manipulation, the heart of the recent court decision, also poses ethical dilemmas. In many instances a totally new organism or therapy is under question. What the short-range and long-range consequences will be and what the unintended and unknown side effects will be are uncertain. Uncertainty does not mean that nothing should be done, however. At the core of scientific discovery and experimentation, uncertainty always exists. Carefully designed scientific means of investigation, meant to minimize risk and benefit the whole person, must be developed. The complexity and intricacy of this field demands caution.

In ethics, caution cannot be translated into stopping scientific investigation or requiring absolute certainty. However, caution does require disciplined and careful analysis, especially because of the possible effects on human beings as individuals and as a society. The possibly grave nature of any errors requires the courage to act for the benefit of others, knowing and respecting the limits of knowledge. Because assessing risks and consequences in this field is not simple does not mean that everything should be halted.

Genetic issues raise other ethical concerns. Improvement in genetic manipulation should not create a greater injustice for those who suffer from genetic anomalies. Concentration on genetics of any sort should not blind society to the socially created and socially induced genetic difficulties that are better resolved in political debate and ethical behavior. Genetic issues are not the sole province of the scientists. Society has too great a stake in these developments not to be included in public debate, policy development, future funding, and implementation. Being a scientist does not give one a monopoly on decision making. To the contrary, the scientist is drawn into a wider decision-making circle by the nature of this work. Further developments in this field can help improve the quality of life to the extent that society realizes the importance of continual research and development and distinguishes its social problems from its medical problems. Blurring these lines will create a false and impossible task for medicine, genetics, and society.

Halting the release of a new organism in a potato field in California reminds all of the necessity to carry on a comprehensive public debate as genetics continues to develop; the importance of careful attention by the scientific community to the possible consequences of this new technology; and the importance of ethical reflection as society asks itself what it wants to become.

Human Reconstruction 26

> The first successful transfer of a
> gene from one animal to another—
> from rabbits to mice and then to their
> offspring—has been achieved by
> biologists. As to applications,
> successful breeding of animals is
> forecast within ten years, with
> medical uses to follow.[1]

In recent years medical technology has moved from being able to repair the human body to being able to remodel the body through genetic reconstruction, which would alter not only an individual but his or her descendants as well. Some of these new capabilities are already practical, and others still futuristic, but if we are to be prepared to introduce these capabilities in an ethical manner, we must consider the principles that should govern this form of activity.

Principles

A basic axiom of medicine has always been the Greek dictum, art perfects nature, which implies that a human being can be healed (or patched up) and developed to maturity but cannot be essentially remade. Today, however, we must face the questions: Is it right for us to become our own creators? Can we and should we remake human nature? Can we hasten the processes of evolution by eliminating our troublesome wisdom teeth or our appendix by genetic engineering? Might we in the future greatly reduce the complexities of the digestive system by a more effective intravenous method? Might we sterilize all human beings and reproduce artificially? Might we also expand the human senses to make it possible for us to see or hear beyond the present or upper range of sight and vision? Might we influence embryological development by drugs to mold the development of the phenotype (the actual body) while not changing the genotype (inherited characteristics)? May we employ genetic engineering to produce any gene combination in the fertilized ovum that we desire, thus creating human beings by "recipe?"

The basic ethical issue is the question of the extent of our dominion over nature. This is a classical way of posing the issue; however, the response to this question by many people is frequently influenced by the Greek image of God as a jealous monarch who becomes angry when Prometheus infringes on his prerogatives. Thus they limit human creativity unnecessarily. Others would view attempts to improve on humankind as either an insult to the work of the creator whose masterpiece is the human being, or as a fatal temptation of pride, because it is a sign that we are trying to replace God.

Today, however, in considering radical human development, we must stress two points: First, God is a generous creator who, in creating us, also called us, by the power of intelligence, to share in his creative power. Consequently, God does not want the talents he has given us to lay fallow, but encourages us to improve on the universe he has made; second, such improvement is possible because we realize that God has made an evolutionary universe in which human beings have been created through an evolutionary process that is not yet complete. Thus God has called us to join with him in bringing the universe to its completion, and in doing this he has not made the human being merely a worker to execute his orders or to add trifling original touches to his own, but he has made the human being a genuine co-worker who is encouraged to exercise real originality.

Discussion

Granted this view however, it does not follow logically that remaking the body on new lines is really the appropriate place for human beings' creativity. We have enough to do remodeling our environment and creating human culture. Moreover, we must realize that our efforts at planning and creating, whether we are planning cities, economies, or human relations, are never very successful. No doubt with greater knowledge we may be able to tidy up some of the business of evolution by removing such vestiges as our wisdom teeth or appendix, if indeed (which is not really known for sure) this would be a real improvement. Someday we may also be able to eliminate genetic disease and even advance human health eugenically. We must remember, however, that our creativity depends on our brain. Any alteration that would injure the brain and hence creativity would indeed be a disastrous mutilation, especially if this were to be transmitted genetically, thus further polluting the gene pool with defects that might be hidden and incalculable.

Generally speaking, our knowledge of our wonderful brain is still in its beginnings. The complexity of the brain is beyond any other system that we can imagine, and this complexity is reduced to a relatively small organ capable of self-development from the embryo and of self-maintenance, but not of self-restoration. Our brain may be near the limit of complexity and integration possible in an organic, living system. In this case any radical improvement may be illusory, while even slight alterations may be very damaging. Thus to say the least, radical attempts to alter the structure of the human brain must be viewed with the utmost caution, since the risk is very high that we will only produce persons of lowered intelligence.

This is certainly not so true of other organ systems, and it is possible to imagine that someday, in other environments, it might become necessary, for example, to replace the human lungs with other ways of obtaining oxygen. In principle it would seem that such changes would be ethical (1) if they gave support to human intelligence by helping the life of the brain and (2) if they did not suppress any of the fundamental human functions that integrate the human personality. Thus alterations that would make it impossible for a human being to sense the external world directly at least as effectively as we do now with our "five senses" would be contrary to well-being of persons and the human community. So would alterations that would make it impossible for human beings to experience the basic emotions, since emotional life is closely related to human intelligence and creativity. Again, alterations that would make human beings sexless and incapable of parenthood would also be antihuman.

Conclusion

In accord with the foregoing, we can draw the following conclusions:

1. Genetic engineering and less radical transformations of the present normal human body would be permissible if they improve rather than mutilate the basic human functions, especially as they relate to supporting human intelligence and creativity. Transformation would be forbidden, however, (a) if human intelligence and creativity are endangered and (b) if the fundamental functions that constitute human integrity are suppressed.

2. Experimental efforts of this radical type must be undertaken with great caution and only on the basis of existing knowledge, not with high risks to the subjects or to the gene pool.

---

1. *Science*, 213 (September 25, 1981): 1488.

Throughout the history of ethics there has been a tendency to treat human sexuality as if it were simply an animal function requiring to be restrained lest it turn human beings into brutes. Modern ethics is insistent that sexuality, as much as any other human function, be specifically humanized or personalized. Human beings should love humanly, just as surely as they should think humanly. In sexual desire and activity, as in all other human functions, we should aim at integration of body-soul dynamics, not a domination or suppression of one by the other. People in health care, because of their role in the community, have the opportunity and responsibility to develop sexual integration in their own lives and to help others develop it as well.

Principles

To build a healthier future it is essential to help people develop a fully integrated and authentic understanding of their sexuality. Health care professionals and health care facilities can play an important role in this developmental task. In order to do so, the following norms must be kept in mind.

The first need in the area of sexuality is to promote balanced programs of sex education. Sound sex education is primarily spiritual and ethical, not only medical, but health care professionals have an essential role to play in it because of its close connection with bodily life. Although many sex education programs today provide excellent biological and psychological information, they also promote a false value system because they neglect the deeper meanings of sexual activity and the responsibilities associated with human love. For instance, sexual education programs that have as an exclusive aim the prevention of pregnancy will cause more harm than good. Concerned people can hardly criticize such programs, however, unless they provide superior ones. A balanced program should begin with helping parents succeed in their natural role as the principal sex educators. Today, many parents suffer either from (1) the predominant influence of secularistic values or from (2) incorrect, distorted religious views that stress negative, repressive aspects of sexual morality that are based on fear, rather than a positive but realistic view based on a true understanding of God's gift of sexuality and of human stewardship.

A sound program of sex education should do the following:

1. Provide for understanding of the unitive-procreative meaning of sexuality in marriage;

2. Provide information on mental hygiene and essential biological facts on sexual differences and equality, lovemaking, intercourse, pregnancy, and birth;

3. Provide information on why people have a need for children and on the problems of sterility and the limits on the right to have children;

4. Provide information on the problems of responsible parenthood in present-day society, natural family planning methods and alternative methods, and ethical evaluation of all birth regulation methods;

5. Explain the rights of the unborn child;

6. Discuss the problems of genetic defects and the supportive attitude toward defective persons developed in the Judeo-Christian tradition; and

7. Consider the problem of homosexuality and similar difficulties in psychosocial development.

Such programs can be considered preventive medicine, since they might go a long way to reduce the frequency or severity of many physiological and psychological problems, but they will not have a widespread effect unless they are also joined to social programs aimed at improving the climate of society.

Discussion

Sound sex education must be based on continuing research and open discussion. When sexual issues are involved, such objectivity is difficult to achieve. It has taken a real struggle on the part of some physicians and nurses to get a hearing for natural methods of delivery and breast-feeding, because such an approach seemed to be an attack on medical "progress." Similarly, in ethical questions dealing with sexual matters, our culture, especially the media, has a strong bias toward voices announcing the coming of new "freedoms" and a suspicion of those who are concerned with explaining the traditional values of family life and enduring love and the disciplined restraint they require. To arrive at an atmosphere in which traditional values can be heard fairly when sexual issues are discussed is extremely difficult. Nonetheless, this atmosphere should be developed.

Health care professionals who play a role in public and social agencies that deal with sexual problems should take care that these agencies do not content themselves merely with more negative means based on a distorted view of human sexuality or a manipulative treatment of young women. Granted that fertility control and responsible parenthood must be an important objective of any such agency, this objective should not be achieved through dehumanizing violence or psychological coercion.

Rather, the principal goal of all such agencies should be to strengthen and promote human dignity and family bonding as basic needs of society. Only in an atmosphere of good family life based on faithful love can coming generations develop a mature, fully integrated human sexuality. As T. S. Eliot wrote:

Lord shall we not bring these gifts to your service?
Shall we not bring to your service all our powers
For life, for dignity, grace and order,
And intellectual pleasures of the senses?
The Lord who created us must wish us to create
And employ our creation again in His service
which is already His service in creating.
For Man is joined spirit and body,
And therefore must serve as spirit and body.
Visible and invisible must meet in His temple;
You must not deny the body!

1. Chorus from the Rock, IX, *Collected Poems of T. S. Eliot, 1909-1950*, (New York: Harcourt Brace, 1971), p. 111.

Sexuality and   28
Sexual Reassignment

Is it ever legitimate to change a person's biological sex? Such surgery, a procedure by which the sexual phenotype of a male is altered to resemble that of a female, or vice versa, is called sexual reassignment. Some physicians believe sexual reassignment is helpful in dealing with the puzzling and painful condition called transsexualism or, more accurately, gender dysphoria syndrome, which is characterized by great anxiety over one's phenotypic sex and socially imposed gender role. Specifically, sexual reassignment involves castration and construction of a pseudovagina for the male and mastectomy and hysterectomy (sometimes also the construction of a nonfunctional pseudopenis and testes) for the female, along with hormonal treatments and psychotherapy.

Ethicists have always admitted that in cases where a child is born with ambiguous genitalia, the parents should raise the child as belonging to that sex in which it is most likely to be able to function best. The reasoning behind this traditional position is that a person must "live according to nature" insofar as this is humanly knowable. Some surgery may be necessary to prepare the child for the "sex where it is most likely to function best."

Recently, however, knowledge of sexual development has vastly increased, and sexual ambiguity is seen as far more complex and common than formerly thought. The biological determination of sex depends on the presence or absence of the Y chromosome in the one-cell zygote that, in the beginning, constitutes the human being. When present, it produces the H-Y antigen as early as the eight-cell stage of development, and the person begins to move toward maleness; otherwise, all zygotes develop as females. All embryos originally have undifferentiated gonads and two sets of sexual ducts, the wolfian and the müllerian, but at seven weeks the male gonads differentiate and begin to produce hormones that destroy the müllerian ducts and cause development of the male genitalia; otherwise the wolfian ducts are absorbed, and the gonads and the müllerian ducts develop into the female sexual system. At the same time the differing hormonal balance in the two sexes causes certain differences in the male and female brains, in particular preparing the female brain to regulate the menstrual cycle.

All these biological determinations are at work before birth. After birth it is probable, but not yet proved, that biophysical events at the unconscious level exist, similar to the imprinting demonstrated in animals, which also promote sexual differentiation, such as the way the mother cares differently for a female or male child. Finally, at the conscious environmental level, the person learns his or her own gender identity and assumes a gender role in society, with the result that in the human population a whole spectrum of conditions exists besides the normal masculine and feminine conditions.

Among these possible abnormalities, homosexuality is a highly varied condition, probably having many etiological factors, in which a person who is phenotypically unambiguously male or female and in no doubt about his or her gender is conscious of greater sexual attraction to those of his or her own sex than to others. Transvestism is a condition in which a person, usually heterosexual, is more comfortable sexually while wearing clothing symbolic of the opposite sex. Transsexualism differs markedly from the aforementioned gender dysphoria syndrome, which is an anxiety, sometimes reaching suicidal depression as the result of the obsessive feeling that one's "real" sex is the opposite of one's phenotypic sex.

The argument of psychotherapists and surgeons who undertake sexual reassignment as a remedy for transsexualism is that the victims find no relief in other therapies, are insistent on surgery even to the point of threatening suicide, and are generally satisfied with its results.

Discussion

Does such reasoning justify sexual reassignment? It seems not, for the following reasons: First, it has not yet been established that the cause of gender dysphoria syndrome is biological. No such cause is evident at the genotypic or phenotypic level, and as yet the evidence is tenuous that the reason transsexuals feel from early in their lives that they have "a soul different from their body" is due to some developmental accident in the central nervous or hormonal systems. At present it remains more probable that the determining causes are at the psychological level of development, although we may admit some biological predispositions. J. K. Meyer went so far as to state, "I have seen any number of men who would like to live as females and vice versa; I have not seen one with a reversal of core gender identity."[1] Consequently, the gender ambiguity in question is primarily psychological and should be treated psychotherapeutically.

Second, when candidates for transsexual surgery are required to undergo psychotherapy in preparation for surgery, many are found to be ambiguous about really wanting it and, in the end, decide against it. Even after surgery they continue to need at least some psychotherapeutic support, although their frequent difficulty in forming stable personal relations makes this follow-up difficult.

Third, although when this type of surgery was first introduced there were some enthusiastic reports of its success, as experience accumulates there is now no solid agreement on whether it does much good. Recently, The Johns Hopkins Medical Center, noted for its leadership in research in the field, announced the suspension of its program for further reassessment.

Fourth, it seems that surgery does not really solve these persons' existential problem, since it does not enable them to achieve sexual normality. Since many of these individuals are somewhat asexual, their problems are not primarily sexual satisfaction, but the relief of the burden of anxiety which can usually be at least considerably lightened by psychotherapy. Moreover, one could question the effort to relieve anxiety through destruction of a basic human function.

For the aforementioned reasons, then, transsexual surgery does not seem to be a legitimate procedure from the ethical perspective. What, then, is the proper therapy? Certainly compassion should be extended to this small but greatly suffering group of human beings, but it should take the form of psychotherapy and personal counseling. The fundamental aim of the therapy should be to restore the person's sense of personal worth. He or she should be helped to realize that today's culture puts exaggerated stress on sexual identity and activity as a determinant of human worth. Thus they should be assisted in escaping their preoccupation with their sexual identity and finding their more fundamental value as a human being.

1. J. K. Meyer, "Psychiatric Considerations in the Sexual Reassignment of Non-Intersex Individuals," *Clinics in Plastic Surgery*, 1(1974): 275-283.

Physicians and other health care professionals often encounter patients who are involved in self-destructive or antisocial behavior that is repulsive or disagreeable. For example, a physician may be asked to treat a married man who, by reason of his many heterosexual and homosexual liaisons, has contracted a venereal disease. The physician, valuing fidelity in marriage, is repelled by the patient and would like "to give him a piece of my mind." The situation may be exacerbated if the physician knows the patient's wife and children. The same reaction might beset other health care professionals as they work with drug addicts and chronic alcoholics. More subtly, these reactions might occur when patients or families wish to have life-supporting means discontinued and the physician wishes to continue them. In these situations, where there is a conflict of values between the health care professional and a patient, the health care professional is usually advised: "Don't be judgmental!"

Principles

As usually interpreted, the slogan "don't be judgmental" means that the health care professional should suppress his or her responses to the patient that arise because of different value systems and should treat the patient as though no conflict existed. For two reasons, though, we submit that this is an unhealthy and self- destructive method of working with patients. First, if the physician or other health care professional tries to suppress value responses, he or she will become ethically schizoid. If one pretends that one can use one set of values in personal life and another in professional life, one will soon disvalue what was formerly valued. Because of the different roles that one has in different areas of human endeavor, some values may be stressed in personal life and others in professional life, but one should never work under the delusion that there is such a thing as "value-free" human activity. Assuming that "value-free" human activity is possible is in itself a value statement that denies most of the values traditional to civilization, the Judeo-Christian culture, and humanism.

Values, standards by which one judges proper or fitting human behavior, reflect what it means to be human and to enter into relationships with other human beings. Values affect every level of human activity: biological, emotional, social, and spiritual. Formed through education, experience, and reflection, values are an important part of one's personality, self-esteem, integrity, and quest for the absolute in which we are all involved. To leave values at home when one goes to the clinic, the laboratory, the operating room, or the intensive care unit is to leave behind a most important part of one's personality.

Second, abandoning values during the hours of professional practice is detrimental to the health care professional because it means that the health care professional will become a slave of other people. Scientists convicted of performing atrocities during World War II offered as their only explanation: "We were only obeying orders." Although this exemplifies the ultimate, it does demonstrate that scientists or physicians who abandon values soon are at the mercy or power of patients, supervisors, politicians, or planners. The example of horror and inhumanity generated through atrocities in World War II made the scientific community realize the danger of pretending that a "value-free science" is possible and demonstrated the effect that such a pretense has on scientists themselves.

Discussion

What, then, is the physician or health care professional to do when working with patients with whom he or she has a value conflict? Should the physician tell the patient to find someone else for treatment, or tell the patient that he will not be worthy of treatment until he leads a better life? Of course not! Rather, there is within the profession of medicine some values that will enable health care professionals to resolve conflicts in a helpful manner. Professions are based on the supposition that people are trying to become better human beings. That is why they come to professionals for help. The professional must value this quest of betterment and realize that it demonstrates the person's basic goodness. To put it another way, when one has a value conflict with another person, each must avoid concluding that the other person is "bad." Rather, each must first realize that the value difference may not be serious or important. Second, even if it is serious or important, we all must realize that the basic goodness of other people is the factor that should dominate relationships. Moreover, we share with a person with whom we disagree the reality that we too are weak and flawed. The professional relationship is not one of superior to inferior, even though the professional has greater skill and knowledge, but rather one of equal to equal because of the basic dignity, destiny, and rights of each person. Valuing the other person, then, should help the health care professional avoid any detrimental or damaging remarks, moralistic reactions, or self-righteous posturing.

Occasionally a serious value conflict may cause the physician to withdraw from serving a patient because the patient requests an action that would compromise the physician's values. If a patient requests a prescription drug that is not medically indicated, or if a patient requests less than proper medical care in order to hasten a relative's death, the physician would have to refuse such petitions. Even in refusing these requests or in withdrawing from service, however, respect for the person in question should not be abandoned.

Another consideration, recognized in every field of human experience as well as in medicine, is that people who engage in destructive behavior are not aided by damaging or vindictive remarks. Beating down another person, or belittling him or her , does not help in overcoming disvalued behavior. Drug abusers and alcoholics do not recover because someone continually berates them. Avoiding damaging remarks and behavior, however, does not mean that the health care professional will never discuss values or detrimental behavior with patients. Indeed, if values have such an important part to play in life, if they influence so much of our behavior and well-being, they should be a factor present in medical diagnosis and prognosis. True, they will usually be in the background of the medical decision-making process, but they should not be eliminated as unimportant. In introducing any discussion of behavior or values with the patient, the health care professional should be guided by the values of medicine, respecting the patient as person.

Conclusion

The essence of medical care concentrates on the particular. No two people are alike. Each encounter with a patient is a new adventure in mutual growth if the professional respects the dignity of the person who comes for help. In this sense, there is a beneficial meaning to the slogan "don't be judgmental."

Masking Ethical Dilemmas 30
in Medicine

> Confusion has risen in some
> professional circles and the public
> mind about the proper role of the
> psychiatrist in medicine and society.
> Being an expert in the science of
> human behavior tends to be equated
> with knowing which behavior is
> morally right. Psychiatrists are
> customarily called in to render
> opinions on what are in fact ethical
> and legal questions in schools, in
> courts, in prisons, and the military.[1]

The above quotation summarizes an article in the *New
England Journal of Medicine*. According to the authors,
primary physicians often call in psychiatrists for consultation,
not realizing that the issues that prompt the call for
consultation are ethical rather than psychiatric. Two serious
difficulties result: (1) "In the process, unfortunately, a moral
consideration of the proposed or expected actions and
considerations of ethical dimensions of the case are often
overlooked or ignored by both primary physician and
psychiatrist;" and (2) "there is a danger in artificially
demarcating physicians' roles in this way...Such an approach
militates against, rather than in favor of, the biopsychosocial
unity of medicine."[2] Although the clinical cases presented in
the article illustrate that the aforementioned difficulties do at
times occur, some ethical guidelines will help both primary
physicians and psychiatrists avoid these difficulties.

Principles

First, physicians must become adept at identifying
medical decisions that have ethical implications. Lo and
Schroeder offer an operational definition of an ethical issue in

medicine: "One that involves a question of what one ought to do, rather than what is usually done or can be done, and that requires a resolution of value choices, as opposed to resolving merely factual or scientific matters."[3] Another word for value is basic human need; thus a value choice involves or affects such things as health, love, life, truth, friendship, freedom, security, self-esteem, the ability to work, the ability to relate to others, the ability to serve others, and other important basic human needs. Hence, whenever a medical decision will affect a basic human need, then the medical decision implies a value or ethical decision. Clearly, few medical decisions of consequence are value free.

Many of the ethical issues that arise in medicine are known to primary physicians as well as to other members of the medical team. Thus, discerning the presence of ethical issues is not always difficult, especially for health care professionals who follow the current literature. In the cases presented in the aforementioned article, the medical team seems to have called in a psychiatrist because there were differences of opinion between physician and patient in regard to the proper procedures. In all three cases, the primary physician attributed the difference of opinion to psychological problems. Actually, the differences were due to differing values. Hence, the first task for the physician or medical team, when differences of opinion arise, is to determine whether they arise because of differing values. If so, an ethical consultation is needed.

Discussion

When physicians and patients disagree, a consultation is not intended to make the patient agree with physician; rather, its purpose is to help the patient make a decision in accord with his or her value system. Hence, ethical consultation must first of all aim at creating an atmosphere in which the patient's freedom is maximized. Unless the patient is freed from coercion and psychological determination, ethical discussion is useless. Until such an opening is achieved, the consultant must strive to keep value discussions at a minimum and not waste time with what seem to be ethical arguments but that in fact are only the expression of emotional conflict. Once the consultant is assured that the patient is sufficiently free to deal with an ethical decision, the next objective is to help the patient arrive at a decision that is at least subjectively good, that is, a decision in accord with the patient's honest conscience. If the consultant is convinced that this decision is not objectively good, that is, in accord with accepted conclusions of medical ethics, then he or she must help form such a decision.

The reason the consultant should first of all help the patient come to a subjectively honest decision is twofold: (1) because the patient always retains primary responsibility for health decisions; and (2) because the proximate norm of all moral decisions is the conscience of the person acting. The task of the consultant, however, does not stop with helping a person arrive at subjectively conscientious decisions. The fact that a decision is honest does not prevent it from being harmful to others or even to the one who makes the decision. Honest mistakes do not injure moral integrity, but they do have consequences that might injure the person or others. Consequently, the consultant cannot be content simply to ratify decisions a patient makes if these decisions will injure the patient or someone else (e.g., in decisions of suicide or murder). In such cases, the consultant must do what is possible to help prevent harm, especially through discussion with the patient, even though the consultant must raise disturbing questions that ultimately go to the root of the patient's value system. Obviously the consultant must be very cautious about disturbing sick people in this manner, yet he or she should have the courage to do so when the patient's own behavior signals that such probing is necessary.

Given the goals of ethical consultation, a variety of competent people might perform the task. The primary physician might be the ethical counselor, the advantage being that the biopsychosocial unity of medical care would be evidenced. A psychiatrist might be called on, the advantage being that he or she would be more adept by training at establishing the atmosphere of freedom that is needed in order to make conscientious ethical decisions. A member of the pastoral care team, trained in counseling, might be called on, the advantage being that he or she is able to help the patient make value decisions in accord with conscience. Perhaps in some cases all three persons might work in unison to help a patient and family reach a difficult decision. In any case, recognition by the medical team that an ethical issue exists and realization of the limited goals of ethical counseling are more important than which health care professional is chosen to act as ethical consultant.

1. Mark Perl and Earl Shelp, PhD, "Psychiatric Consultation Masking Moral Dilemmas in Medicine," *New England Journal of Medicine*, 307(1982): 618-621.
2. Perl and Shelp, p. 619.
3. Bernard Lo and Stephen A. Schroeder, "Frequency of Ethical Dilemmas in a Medical Inpatient Service," *Archives of Internal Medicine*, 141(1981) 1062-1064.

Case Study: Disagreeing With a Full Code Order. Ms. Doris Winn, a staff nurse with two years' experience in a cardiac care unit, strongly disagreed with Dr. Cunningham's full code order for Mr. Chester Saukin, an 87-year old retired farmer with a history of three myocardial infarctions and three years of cardiac failure. Ms. Winn believed that Mr. Saukin was ready to die, since he had told her that was all he wanted. When she told Dr. Cunningham this, he simply walked away from her. She knew he always ordered full codes for all his patients. Ms. Winn understood also that legally she had to do the full code, but she thought it would be very hard for her.

Using case studies is a helpful educational method in medical ethics. With this method, people interested in medical ethics are able to apprehend ethical issues, to apply their value systems, to gain some insight into balancing rights and responsibilities, and to sharpen skills needed in solving day-to-day problems. When solving case studies, however, one of the most important ethical questions is often overlooked, how to ensure that the situation that gave rise to the ethical issue or dilemma does not occur again.

Principles

The case cited offers a good illustration. One could get so involved in determining the rights of Chester Saukin, the validity and sincerity of his request to be allowed to die, the obligation of Dr. Cunningham to preserve life, his responsibility to respect the other members of the health care team, and recourse for Doris Winn that one might overlook the significant question: How to avoid this situation in the future? This question is founded on the experience that many ethical questions can be foreseen and handled in advance if well-designed policies are formulated and applied. The wisdom and indeed the use of medical ethics is found not only in solving ethical problems but in obviating their reoccurrence. Problems that concern the use of cardiopulmonary resuscitation, for example, could occur continually in a health care facility caring for aging patients if a well-thought-out policy that gives general procedures does not exist. In times past, openly discussing controversial or difficult ethical decisions in medical and health care, especially decisions that might occur if there were danger of death, was not common. Today, however, greater openness and ability to face such issues is common among health care workers and administrators. To date, however, although some health care facilities have formulated policies on a few ethical issues, no general awareness exists on the need for this type of managerial initiative to foresee and avoid difficult ethical problems.

Discussion

In general, clearcut policies should be developed for three kinds of recurring ethical problems:

1. Problems that arise as a result of differing opinions between health care professionals concerning rights and responsibilities in patient care. Often, such problems are described as problems in human relations, but they are serious ethical problems as well. A policy addressing this potential problem area must incorporate a method of honest and open dialogue between health care professionals. Simply saying "that's the way we've always done it" or walking away from the confrontation, as Dr. Cunningham did, will not solve the ethical and emotional question. For teamwork to flourish, a team leader is needed. Leadership among professionals, however, must be founded on mutual respect and willingness to discuss relevant issues that contribute to quality patient care.

2. Problems that arise in regard to informing patients of their rights and responsibilities. In this general category are

included such issues as obtaining informed consent for surgical and medical procedures, and notifying patients in advance about payments for services and criteria needed to qualify for charitable care. In general, obviating this type of ethical problem requires clear and proper instruction by the physician or a representative of the physician or the facility. Negligence in regard to obtaining informed consent has been documented, so policy statements should be formulated with this tendency in mind. Explaining monetary responsibilities in advance will obviate some of the unjust criticism that arises if these responsibilities are not clearly apprehended.

3. Problems that admit of varying solutions but for which there should be a definite procedure in seeking a solution. For example, whether to allow a patient to die cannot be determined in advance, but the questions that should be asked, the people who should be consulted, and the method of involving the patient and family members in the proper decision should be outlined in a policy. The use of cardiopulmonary resuscitation, declaration of brain death, permission for transplantation, procedures in triage situations, how to inform parents of genetically affected children, and how to present options for treatment to chemically dependent patients are problems that fit into this category of concern.

Who should formulate these policies and state the proper protocols? Because most of the situations that have been described take place in health care facilities, the governing body is responsible for making sure that ethical policies are formulated. Employees in various health care specialities should actually formulate the policies for two reasons: (1) they have the knowledge and experience necessary for effective policy formulation; and (2) they should be interested in improving the ethical effectiveness of their profession. Thus in every health care facility there should be an ethics committee composed of various health care professionals, responsible to the administration, whose task is to formulate policies that will obviate ethical problems.

Such committees are not decision-making groups; they do not nor should they sit in judgment over fellow health care professionals. Rather, they have a specific educational task that should be carried out in the following manner: (1) investigating the areas of conflict in the health care facility that need attention; (2) working with people involved to formulate policies and presenting the policies to the administration for approval; (3) designing educational programs to help concerned health care professionals apply the policies carefully and effectively.

Opting for judicious policies to obviate recurring ethical dilemmas is not a form of neo-utopianism. Rather, it is simply applying sound principles of management to important problems of human concern.

Addiction or   32
Chemical Dependency

Although it is not often listed as a cause of death, chemical addiction is a serious cause of health disorders among people in the United States. More detrimental than its physiological effects, however, are the familial, social, and spiritual harms that result from chemical addiction. Almost everyone has a loved one whose addiction to alcohol or drugs is a cause of deep concern. Because chemical addiction disposes for, and causes, so much illness and suffering, a few thoughts from the ethical point of view concerning this phenomenon are in order.

Although its development is not fully understood, one component of chemical dependency is physical pleasure. In the face of difficulty, tension, or frustration, the chemically dependent person runs away from the loss of normal satisfaction and achievement by indulging in the physical pleasure and relaxation of the addicting experience. The search for pleasure alone does not constitute addiction, however. Rather, the increasing sense of guilt and helplessness that accompanies each overindulgence intervenes with the pleasurable result, so that the incipient addict begins to indulge not for the sake of pleasure itself, but to blot out the guilt and remorse for the consequences of previous indulgences. Furthermore, this vicious circle is reinforced by the use of psychological coping mechanisms, such as rationalization and denial, which victims find necessary to assist in this suppression of guilt and pain. Thus victims become increasingly unable to perceive the real consequences of their behavior. Extensive research shows that although causes of chemical addiction are often physiological, the psychological component remains essential, so that persons who lack this component can sometimes use even so highly addictive a drug as heroin without exhibiting the typical features of addiction.

Principles

Is one personally responsible for addiction? On the one hand, therapists speak of addiction as a "disease" in order to reduce its moral opprobrium and to achieve a more sympathetic attitude on the part of nonaddicts. On the other hand, an important part of therapy is to get addicts to accept moral responsibility for the harm they have done themselves and others through addiction. This ambiguity can be cleared up if two points are kept in mind. First, chemical dependency is always a psychological disease, since it involves an abnormal behavior pattern accompanied by the neurotic coping mechanisms already described. It is also a physiological disease because it sometimes produces physiological dependency and usually produces widespread organic changes that greatly aggravate the condition. Second, voluntary and free acts must be distinguished. Addictive behavior is voluntary because it proceeds from an inner desire, but it always involves a restriction of freedom, since the desire is compulsive and the addict becomes less able to perceive alternatives of action or to choose among them. In times of addictive need the addict's practical conscience is concerned totally with the need for a drink or a fix. He or she acts voluntarily and compulsively, but without free choice.

Hence, actual consumption of addictive substances by addicts is seldom in itself a morally culpable act because of diminished freedom, and the guilt felt afterward is mainly unrealistic and neurotic. Although there may be some moral awareness of future difficulty when one starts using a potentially addictive substance, even the acquisition of addiction often proceeds so gradually and subtly that it is difficult to judge that the addict knowingly and deliberately chooses addiction. Nevertheless, it would be a mistake to think that all guilt experienced by addicts is illusory or neurotic. If it were, it would be hard to explain why admission of responsibility has proved so important a part of therapy. In sum, the most realistic and productive way to express responsibility for addiction is to say that the addicted person has the obligation to ask and receive help from others, since therapy cannot be effective until the addict accepts help.

Discussion

Health care professionals' ethical responsibility concerning addiction may be summarized as follows:

1. Realizing that addiction causes so much illness and sorrow, health care professionals must acquaint themselves thoroughly not only with the nature and therapy of addiction, but also with the ways to persuade addicts to accept treatment, the treatment centers to which they can be referred, and the ways to support them in their efforts. Moreover, families and friends of addicts should be persuaded to treat addicts as victims of illness rather than as morally responsible delinquents. Helping the family of the addict to be fair, but not overprotective, is an important goal for persons in health care.

2. Health care professionals should be aware that they themselves have a chemical dependency rate higher than people in other occupations. Whatever the causes of this proclivity, individuals should develop a life style with the proper psychological and spiritual means to overcome this tendency. Adequate and enriching relaxation and sensitive concern for others should be the bedrock of this life style.

3. Perhaps an even more effective way for health care professionals to combat chemical addiction is through preventive measures. They can play an important role in combating the drug culture mentality in the United States. According to this mentality, every pain, every sorrow or frustration, can be overcome with a pill, potion, or injection of some kind. Pharmaceutical firms constantly publicize drugs, such as tranquilizers, and health care professionals often are used by such firms to promote unnecessary drug use. Responsible professionals will not share in this promotion, because they realize that human pain, frustration, and sorrow cannot be simply suppressed. Human beings grow as persons by facing and working through the difficulties of life realistically as free people, not by running away from them and becoming slaves to a pleasure ethos. In this view, we are not proposing an exaggerated stoicism as the ideal of ethical behavior. Rather, we are calling for a realistic effort to overcome the sorrow and suffering of life through relaxation and diversion, such as contemplation, music, and

companionship, which renew rather than destroy the human personality. Alcoholics Anonymous, which has led the way to the most successful methods of therapy for chemical dependency, has always emphasized that the addict cannot recover unless he or she reaches out to a higher power, is willing to repair damage done to loved ones, and serves one's neighbor. There is a message here as well for those of us who are not yet wholly addicted.

Determining Death 33

Many ethical decisions in medicine are based on a determination of the fact of death, such as when to remove life-support systems, when to inform a family that a loved one is no longer living, and when to allow an organ to be taken from a cadaver. Hence, in order to make sound ethical decisions in health care, one must have an accurate concept of human life and human death.

When biologists speak of the death of any living organism, they refer to that inevitable and critical moment when an organism ceases to function as a specific, unified, homeostatic system and becomes instead a disorganized collection of heterogeneous chemical substances. Sometimes, even after the moment of death, some merely physiological functions continue in a disorganized manner. The death of a human person is like any other death and is determined by various signs that the unifying life force (the soul) is no longer informing the body even though some isolated organ or cell function may continue.

Principles

What are the signs that the unifying life force is still present? We can be certain death has not yet occurred as long as a person can communicate through speech or gesture. When such communication ceases, we can only judge by signs that are no longer distinctly and specifically human, such as physiological functions of the heart or lungs. Yet we do not dare to conclude quickly that death has occurred merely because specifically human signs are no longer evident, as becomes very clear when we observe someone wake from sleep or coma.

Consequently, we are morally obliged to treat anybody who is apparently human (even in the fetal state) as a human being with human rights until we are sure that the body has become so disorganized that it no longer retains its source of unity. To know that the source of unity is absent, we must be reasonably sure of three things: (1) that the body does not now exhibit specific human behavior; (2) that it will not be able to function humanly in the future; and (3) that it no longer has even a radical capacity for human functions because it has lost the basic structures required for human unity. This third condition is required because medical experience has shown that persons who have been in prolonged apparently irreversible coma have sometimes recovered full human consciousness. Moreover, resuscitation is possible as long as the radical structures of the human organism remain and the causes that inhibit their normal function can be removed. (This is why some speculate that in the future the human body may be able to be frozen and revived centuries later.)

There is no reason to deny that after true human death some cells or even organs of the human body may for a time (perhaps indefinitely if artificially supported) continue to exhibit some life functions that are not those of the human organism as a unified entity. Hence the essential point about determining human death is not to decide whether any life (cell action) is present, but whether *human life* in the most radical sense of a unified human person is still present.

Discussion

Certainly, some signs of human death were always easy to identify. If rigor mortis or putrefaction occurs, then even nonprofessionals are able to recognize that the human organism is irreversibly destroyed. Other less conclusive signs of human death were the absence of breathing and heartbeat because it was known that heart and lung function might sometimes be revived by resuscitation. When resuscitation efforts fail, death is judged certain, and physicians pronounce the patient dead on the basis of clinical evidence certifying the time of death for legal purposes such as inheritance. Thus cessation of spontaneous heart and lung function became known as the *clinical* signs of death.

In recent times, two developments have led to the proposal of a new set of clinical signs for determining the fact of human death. First, machines have been perfected that artificially aid or sustain the function of the heart and lungs. Such artificially sustained heart and lung action is not certain proof that human life still remains, but as long as heart and lungs are sustained artificially it is impossible to verify the traditional signs of human death. Clearly, one may be able to maintain heart and lung action, at least temporarily, even after the source of unity is no longer present. We know that the heart completely separated from the body can continue to beat, and tissues in a test tube can continue to exhibit some residual life if nourished by an appropriate solution. Therefore the question arises: Can other clinical signs be used, not to constitute a new definition of death, but as alternative means to establish the same essential fact, namely, that the principle of human unified activity is no longer present?

The second, and perhaps more important, reason for seeking new clinical signs of death has been the recent advancement of techniques of organ transplantation, especially of the kidney and heart. Such transplantations are more likely to be successful if the organs are retrieved from a body through which blood is circulating. Hence surgeons prefer to keep the body of a "dead" donor "alive" on a respirator.

How, then, is it possible to be sure that the donor is in fact dead if the traditional signs, cessation of heart and lung function cannot be verified? Brain death criteria may be employed because brain function is an even more fundamental sign that the unifying life source is present than is the function of heart and lungs. We can posit the continuing life of a person if the heart and lung functions are temporarily supplied by machines, as happens in open heart surgery, if the brain is still able to function. But if the brain cannot function and this condition is irreversible, then there is no way we can reverse the disintegration of the brain and no way we can posit that the principle of unity, the life-giving force (the soul), is still present. Medical research demonstrates that if the brain has ceased to function irreversibly, then it is being destroyed because blood is not circulating effectively, even though the brain may not have lost all signs of cellular activity! Although it is not our purpose to settle any of these differences of opinion in regard to medical signs of brain death, it is our ethical conclusion that when total and irreversible function of brain activity is clinically proven, the person in question is dead because the human form (soul) is no longer able to inform the matter.

Notice that the clinical signs for brain death should be utilized only when a transplant is anticipated and organs are to be harvested from the corpse of the dead person. In other circumstances the life-support systems should be removed and the traditional clinical signs utilized, namely, the irreversible cessation of heart and lung function. Ethically speaking, in most cases it is an abuse to keep a person on life-support systems until brain death occurs if a transplant is not anticipated.

Would it be possible to declare a person dead if only the higher neocortical centers, on which it appears human thought processes depend, ceased to function? Some are willing to defend this view on the grounds that the specifically human functions are destroyed when neocortical function is lost irreversibly.[2] But it seems that this opinion is medically and ethically unacceptable. Today, it is generally recognized that the brain is a system of subsystems that are interdependent. Although it is possible to localize such functions as speech and sight in particular parts of the brain, this is not proof that only one part is involved in the functions or even that it is its primary center, since inhibition of a merely secondary or auxiliary part of a system may impede a particular function. Thus death should not be certified as long as patients are able to maintain spontaneous breathing and heart beat, since this constitutes strong evidence that the brain as the seat of radical unity of the human body is still functioning in a unifying manner, even though it is evident that higher functions are impaired.

1. Gaetano Molinari, MD, "Review of Clinical Criteria of Brain Death;" *Brain Death: Interrelated Medical and Social Issues*, (New York: New York Academy of Sciences, 1978) p. 62-70.
2. Robert Rizzo and Paul Yonder, "Definition and Criteria of Clinical Death," *Linacre Quarterly* 40(1973): 223-233.

Do Not Resuscitate! 34

   In hospitals, long term care facilities, and other health
care institutions, cardiopulmonary resuscitation or "code
blue" calls are routine for the young as well as for the old.
Increasingly, because of lack of clear information, such calls
are questioned by the nursing staff that care for the patients
on a daily basis, by the competent patient who does not want
to be resuscitated or by family members who wonder if
resuscitation is beneficial for their loved ones. Such
questioning raises difficult moral issues. Is medical
negligence involved; are patients' rights respected? Our
purpose is to dispel some of the misunderstanding in regard to
ethical care for patients by contrasting the ethical norms for
"code" and "no code" orders.
   "Code blue" calls, or cardio-pulmonary resuscitation,
bringing together a group of highly skilled people around a
patient's bed, are designed to "save" a person's life by
administering quality care at a particular moment of crisis in
the patient's life. The health care team working on a patient in
cardiac distress attempts to resolve a difficult medical
situation in order that other medical problems from which the
patient suffers might be cured or alleviated so that the patient
might return home and resume some, if not all, functions of
normal life. The code blue procedure is designed to help a
patient live. Moral questions arise when the possibility of life is
no longer present, when the patient is suffering from a
terminal disease and death is imminent, and when the patient,
family member, or legal guardian asks that a "no-code" order
be written. In these situations, the physician may feel that a
written no-code order speaks of medical negligence, is a
possible indicator of malpractice, and is legally dangerous.
The nurses and other health care providers may see the
physician as cold, unresponsive to the patient's needs, and
aloof if he or she does not respond to a no-code request or
look upon him or her as irresponsible and insensitive if a no-
code order is given too easily, as though the health care team
were giving up on the patient.

Principles

A no-code order, like a code blue call, should be looked upon as a medical judgment made by those responsible for medical care. The decision to code or no-code is made in light of the patient's values and the status of his or her health. Thus, a no-code order is given by the physician in light of what is good, sound medical treatment. In a no-code situation, unlike the code blue call, the patient is judged to be dying and prolongation of life is an ethically extraordinary and nonobligatory procedure. Clearly, in some cases a code blue call would be an unnecessary burden for the patient or a useless medical procedure that would not help the patient return to a more beneficial situation. If either of these judgments is made by the physician, a no-code order may be written. Contrary to the notion that a no-code order is an indication of medical negligence, such an order might in fact be medically indicated as the proper kind of care for this dying patient. A no-code order, then, may well be a protection against overaggressive treatment.

A no-code order, like all other medical orders, must be communicated effectively. A clear, legible statement should be placed on the patient's chart by the attending physician. Such communication enables the nursing staff and other health care providers to give continuous and quality care to the patient that is in line with the decisions made by the patient, family members, or legal guardians in conjunction with the physician. Supportive care for the patient's dying and true palliative care can be realized only when the physician and the health care team communicate and cooperate. In the same spirit of good medical practice, such an order should be reviewed periodically to ensure that the patient's status has not changed and that such an order is still medically indicated. Often, consultation with another physician or a request that the hospital ethics committee review the ethical dimension of the decision can ensure that an appropriate decision has been made for the patient.

A no-code order also respects the patient's physical and spiritual values which are at stake in the dying process. Recognizing that this patient cannot be "saved" by medical science, one respects the limits of the physical realities while at the same time allowing the spiritual beliefs about life after death and the importance of the person as an embodied spirit to be fulfilled. Dying is a part of the life process for each individual. Helping a patient to die well, and providing medical care that alleviates pain while not giving unnecessary or nonobligatory care, can be medically indicated and consistent with the dignity of each individual.

Discussion

In light of the above statements, who decides for or against a no-code order and when is that decision made? It is the physician's responsibility, with consultation when necessary, to ascertain that a patient is terminally ill and that death is imminent. It is his or her responsibility to indicate the medical treatment (possibly simply palliative) most appropriate in this case.

Once such a decision has been made, the physician must obtain permission for such a course of action. If the patient is competent, the patient and the physician should make such a decision together. If the patient is incompetent, the family members or legal guardian must be consulted. When the physician initiates such an action, the patient or the family may not accept it and may request that everything possible be done to keep the patient alive. Simply ignoring the family's decisions would not be ethical for the physician. But a request made by the family does not necessarily have to be the final word. The physician's skills in such a "counseling" situation are important. Perhaps the family may not understand that (1) resuscitation for moribund people suffering from multiple pathologies is seldom successful; or (2) resuscitation occasionally leaves a patient with only vegetative function; or (3) successful resuscitation implies that the patient will be able to survive the present illness.

On the other hand, the patient, when competent, or the family or legal guardian of the incompetent patient may request that there be no resuscitation. When such a request is received, the physician must give an accurate picture of the patient's condition vis-a-vis his or her illness or death. When death is imminent and the responsible parties have come to a mutual decision, then a no-code order may be written as described above.

Other situations may arise. A competent patient who is not dying may request that a no-code order be given. Ethical conflict will arise here if the physician sees resuscitation as a way of prolonging life in a beneficial manner even though the patient sees resuscitation or prolonging life as a burden. In conflict cases, the physician may perceive continued involvement as a participation in the patient's suicide. The transfer of this patient to another physician's care in an unprejudiced manner is permissible. Usually ethical conflicts can be resolved through consultation with a third party; for example, a member of the pastoral care department.

If the family of an incompetent patient wishes a no-code order written, the physician will usually be able to agree with this request. But, if a conflict arises in regard to the order and it cannot be resolved, the court should be consulted. Although some useful decisions have resulted from such conflicts, for example, the Quinlan and Conroy decisions; in general, involvement of the courts should be kept to a minimum. The main reason for avoiding the courts is to keep ethical decision making where it belongs: in the physician-family relationship.

Conclusion

A no-code order is medically indicated in some cases in health care institutions. It is not an indication of medical negligence nor does it indicate that normal care for a dying patient will be overlooked or lessened. As in all medical decisions, the patient, the family, and the physician should cooperate and communicate before any no-code order is written.

Evaluating In Vitro Fertilization: 35
A Methodology
Principles

     When preparing a scientific protocol, the most important part of the endeavor is asking the right questions. If the wrong questions are posed, then the project will fail, even though the scientist might find the answers to the questions posited. When preparing an ethical evaluation, the situation is similar. One must be careful to pose the proper, the comprehensive, the right questions, or one certainly will reach an erroneous or only partially valid conclusion. This methodological truth is illustrated clearly in the ethical evaluation of in vitro fertilization (IVF). If IVF is successful, a married couple who have been infertile are able to have a child of their own. Insofar as the parents of the child are concerned, then, the result of IVF is good. But this limited view of the situation does not allow the conclusion that IVF is an ethical good. Simply because one result is good does not imply that the matter in question is good under every aspect. For an action to be judged ethically good it should be good from every point of view. In addition to the parents' benefit, then, other questions concerning the effects on the child and society, as well as the nature of the generative act, must be considered before an accurate ethical evaluation of IVF can be offered. What are the right questions that should be posed in order to evaluate IVF properly? The following interrelated questions seem to be essential for an evaluation of IVF.

Discussion

1. When does life begin?
   Significance: If human life begins at fertilization, then IVF is experimentation on a human being and should follow the norms of that type of research. Moreover, discarded zygotes or embryos lost in unsuccessful implantations, at present a

foreseen possibility of IVF, would be human. Steptoe reported that out of 150 attempts to implant human embryos, only four actually were successful and only one was carried to term.[1] Knowingly and willingly wasting human beings is unethical. On the other hand, if there is evidence that human life does not begin until after implantation, then IVF would not be unethical because only animal life would be present. The following query sums up this aspect of the issue: Is the zygote human life with potential or potential human life?

2. How should children be brought into the world?
Significance: Pleasure, a disposition for love, and procreation of children are natural components of the act of sexual intercourse. Today, human beings have the power to separate artificially these elements of the act. Thus it is comparatively simple to ensure through intervention in the natural generative processes, either that the procreation of children will not occur even though persons join in sexual intercourse, or that it will occur, obviating sexual intercourse. Although we have the power to do these things, do we have the *right*? Because a couple is infertile, do they have the right, with the aid of scientists, to circumvent the natural process of generation? Or are the creative powers that people share with God limited in such a way that they should stop short of interfering with natural processes such as the generation of new human beings, even though it is clear that a substitute method for the natural process can be found? Clearly, we have the right to modify our bodily entity so that natural actions are more aptly performed. But do we have the right to change our bodily entity so that natural actions are eliminated, the same results being achieved through artificial means?

3. What results (consequences) will IVF have on parents, children, and society?
Significance: Bonding (effective love) arises from intimate physical and emotional contact between parents and children. Would the result of less physical and emotional contact in the generation of in vitro children weaken family bonding? Will in vitro children be looked on as possessions rather than as persons with their own rights and destinies? Will they be as secure as natural children? In

an ethical evaluation, in order to understand the nature and consequences of a particular action, it is sometimes helpful to ask, "What if everyone does it all the time?" What effect would there be on society and the family if the fertilization and even gestation of all children were achieved in a wholly artificial manner? The family has had a dramatic effect on the evolution of the human species.[2] Would the development of the family and thus the progress of society be weakened by IVF? Have the potential effects of such far-reaching changes in the process of human generation on children, parents, and society been evaluated?

4. To which projects should research efforts of medicine and science be directed?
   Significance: The resources of society are limited and should be directed toward projects that will benefit as many people as possible and that will alleviate serious health problems. Is infertility a serious health problem? Is IVF the best method for treating it? Have the efforts invested in IVF to date justified the results? Would a sufficient number of people benefit from IVF to justify the time and energy necessary to develop it from the comparatively unsuccessful process that it is today to the point where it is more dependable as a means of generation?[3]

Conclusion

IVF is but one of the many forthcoming medical procedures capable of drastically modifying human activities and relationships. Genetic surgery and gene splicing are on the horizon, and they too will have great influence on the human genotype and phenotype and thus on the family and society. Are such procedures a beneficial and wise use of our limited resources. Only when a procedure is good from all points of view can it be declared ethically acceptable.

1. Patrick Steptoe, "Reimplantation of a Human Embryo with a Subsequent Tubal Pregnancy." *The Lancet* (1976): 880-882.
2. Ed Johanson, *Lucy, The Beginning of Mankind*. (New York: Simon & Schuster, 1981).
3. J. Biggers, "In Vitro Fertilization and Embryo Transfer in Human Beings." *New England Journal of Medicine*, 304(1981): 336-342.

Surrogate Parenting

The results of modern medical technology fascinates most people, especially when it is used to promote life, cure people of formerly incurable diseases, or provide a child to people who for some reason are not able to have a child of their own. It is easy for the consequences of these procedures, however, to cover the intricate ethical issues that arise regardless of the "good" consequence of the activity. Such was the case with the birth of Christopher Ray Stiver, Jan. 10, 1983, in Lansing, Michigan. Christopher raised many ethical questions because he was not "normal." The child of a surrogate mother, he was microcephalic, perhaps mentally retarded, had a severe infection, needed immediate medical attention, and was not what his "parents" wanted. Although surrogate parenting promises hope for some women who are not able or who do not wish to conceive and carry their own child, it also raises serious ethical questions for society. The following questions must be evaluated carefully if we are to make an ethical assessment of surrogate parenting.

Principles

The first question strikes at the core of social existence — the central place of the family. The family is envisioned as a central place for identity, socialization, intimacy, and affection in society. Should this be threatened or changed by such methods of parenting? What would happen to the place of the child in society if we select children based on any number of variables considered in the selection process of insemination and fertilization? What are the long-term effects on the surrogate parents and their child? Should our basic values in regard to family be changed by this medical possibility?

A second set of questions involves sex, sexuality, and reproduction. These values are united in the person. Previous examples of their separation have led to all sorts of destructive dualisms that are recognized as unhealthy. Is heterologous insemination and surrogate parenting another contemporary example of this dualistic nemesis? Can we really separate one's sexuality from the reproductive concerns of a society? Granted, we may be able to do this scientifically and conceptually, but should we? What will be the long-term results of such a separation to the person and to society? There is no question that parenting one's own genetic child is a value and that sterility and fertilization problems need medical attention, but does surrogate parenting resolve these difficult medical issues or only mask the need to deal with these issues more carefully? Does a couple have a *right* to children by any means? Are children products, the result of parental rights, secured in such a fashion, or are they a gift? When one uses the sperm or the womb of another person for the purpose of having children, is one subtly using another person as a means rather than as an end? Is payment for these services a breakdown of healthy attitudes about family, sexuality, women, and babies?

Third, and related to the above questions, is the question of heterologous insemination (AID). There are legal and ethical difficulties with this technique, as evidenced by Christopher's birth and subsequent need for medical attention. Who decides? Does sperm donation create an obligation to the child, especially if the child is not what the father wanted? What happens, as it has in other cases, when the mother refuses to "give up" the child to the contracting father? Does AID compromise or cheapen the beauty of sexual activity and the basis of family and love through which children are conceived? What happens to the child when there are complications that call into question who the father really is? Although AID may provide a technical way around some pregnancy issues, does it threaten the life of the child in the long run?

Discussion

A 1983 article in the *New England Journal of Medicine* raises another question. What is the relationship between the mother and the fetus in the prenatal experience? The authors state, "Parental recognition of the fetal form is a fundamental element in the later parent-child bond." What happens when this is not present? Verney contends that the relationship between the mother and the fetus is critical to later relationships in family life and in some cases an important clue to later psychological issues.[2] Although both these findings need more research, can surrogate parenting continue when such critical issues are in the balance? Such research may raise serious questions about the ethics of such reproductive practices, especially when distancing is required by the surrogate mother during pregnancy.

The final series of questions deals with contemporary attitudes about children. With great technological know-how we have not created a something, but a person, a child. This strikes at the core of the issue—baby producing, which is a human event, not an industrial feat. The tragedy of Christopher is that he came into the world helpless, greatly desired by his parents, but with no assurance of his welfare or continued care. His medical problems are serious, but he is not a monster—he is simply impaired, unwanted, not exactly what had been ordered or hoped for, almost discarded as a "poor-quality production." These phrases disturb, are harsh, but they point to the underlying issues of artificial reproduction. Can society tolerate, indeed survive, if its children are not wanted because they *are*, but are wanted only because they fulfill parental desire and physical expectations? It must be realized that even in his fragile condition, Christopher is a person and not a thing.

The healthy child born in such circumstances brings joy and awe that medical science can and does help a couple realize an important dream, but such success can mask the ethical dilemmas that remain. Christopher's birth reminds us that medical advances are for the protection and improvement of human life in all its dimensions. To forget this, because we are normally pleased with the results, will prevent us from making sound ethical judgments.

1. J. C. Fletcher and M. L. Evans, "Maternal Bonding in Early Fetal Ultrasound Examinations," *New England Journal of Medicine* 308(1983): 392-393.
2. Thomas Verney and John Kelly, *The Secret Life of The Unborn Child* (New York: Delta Books, 1982).

Cases and Articles

Elizabeth Bouvia, a twenty-six-year-old quadriplegic cerebral palsey victim, admitted herself into the psychiatric ward of Riverside General Hospital, Riverside, CA, on Sept. 3, 1983. She requested that physicians provide her with analgesics to relieve pain as she starved to death.[1] Her case presents a complex ethical dilemma wherein a number of ethical principles conflict.

Principles

Four major areas of concern intersect in this case. First, the well-established principle of patient autonomy is at issue. Ethics, medicine, and law have long respected a patient's right to accept or refuse treatment. Following the competent adult's decision has been a fundamental norm of medical ethics. Questions arise in Bouvia's case on whether she is competent; however, neither a critical illness nor her decisions are accurate indicators of her competency. Whether a person understands the illness, the consequences of his or her decision, and the alternatives available is more indicative of competency than whether a certain treatment is chosen. Autonomy, however, is not absolute.

A second issue is the role that the quality of life plays in ethical decisions. Elizabeth Bouvia has stated: "The quality of my life is over." Her perception of her total dependency on others led her to request aid in her death wish. Some would respond to her wish with a statement based on some form of the "sanctity of life." Life is sacred and can never be taken because of a transcendent or religious dimension. Some would even include the sanctity of all life—plant, animal, and human—as a reason for not allowing life to be taken. In its most extreme form, such a view would absolutize the maintenance of bodily or physiological functioning. "Quality of life" arguments run a similarly wide gambit. Some would argue that the loss of mobility, or the loss of mental functioning, or the inability to have a "useful" existence is cause to terminate life. Others in this line of argument would ask whether one can realize the important relational and higher function of life, such as love of God, love of neighbor, and social existence. Either side of this argument can foster an oversimplification of complex ethical issues (see chapter 19).

A third area of concern lies in one's perception of medicine. The primary principle behind much of medical ethics has been that the medical profession should first of all "do no harm." All treatments should benefit the patient, benefit being defined not solely in terms of cure, but also in terms of care, especially for dying patients. To request that health care professionals participate in actions that promote unnecessary destruction has generally been seen as unethical. Many examples abound: prescriptions for illicit drugs; killing prisoners sentenced to capital punishment; unethical experimentations on human subjects; compliance with the wishes of guardians that harm patients for whom they are making decisions.

This particular principle raises issues in terms of active and passive euthanasia. The critical point in these cases is not whether one performs or omits an action, but the broader issue of how the action or omission relates to the patient's condition. Not to resuscitate the dying cancer victim is very different from not resuscitating the thirty-year-old cardiac arrest victim not suffering from terminal illness. Likewise, to administer morphine to the terminal lung cancer patient to relieve unnecessary pain that hastens a person's death due to toxicity is ethically different than administering an overdose to the patient who has a life-threatening disease that is not terminal. Questions of euthanasia in Elizabeth Bouvia's case rest on this distinction. Indeed, she has a life-threatening illness that, at this point, is not terminal. She is not about to die. Is aiding her death an active and therefore unethical form of euthanasia because one arbitrarily hastens her death, or is it a passive form of euthanasia in the sense of allowing a disease to take its normal course and to respect her dying as a "normal" or "last" act of her living?

The final issue is the social consequence of Elizabeth Bouvia's activity. Although personal freedoms, autonomy in choices, are important aspects of each individual's life, no person's choices are made in a total vacuum. Each person's choices have some effect on a broader population. To argue for pure autonomy leads one into untenable positions in which no social responsibilities or social benefits exist. Personal autonomy is not absolute and has been circumscribed by medicine, law, and ethics, where issues affect more than the individual.

Discussion

Society at large, medicine, health care professionals, and other disabled individuals will be affected by the decision made in this case. Other disabled citizens, medicine, and society have legitimate interests in Elizabeth Bouvia's decisions, and their concerns are neither necessarily intrusive nor irrelevant.

Elizabeth Bouvia's request challenges contemporary society. More than ever before, medicine has the technological capability of keeping alive those whose physical and mental impairments would have ended in death at birth or early in life. How these people are treated, how their choices are respected, and how society adapts to their needs is crucial. How her case is handled is crucial to the future directions our society takes in dealing with the disabled, and how society deals with care for the disabled should not be arbitrary.

In addition, this case raises the issue of quality of life in an acute manner. A vitalistic or absolutist stand, which requires that "respect for life" mean the maintenance of physical life alone, is untenable. The quality of Elizabeth Bouvia's life is significant. This quality of life, however, is a challenge to the social construction of reality, which is a significant element of all our lives. It is not enough to say that ethical imperatives exist against euthanasia or suicide. Rather, society is challenged to find ways to include the lives of the physically and mentally disabled in a meaningful fashion. Bouvia's case challenges not only medicine in terms of her care, but the social myths that promote independence, self-sufficiency, and individualism as a primary model of full human life.

Finally, which concern should take precedence? This is not an easy question. No one of the concerns claims sole priority. Elizabeth Bouvia's case is complicated because all principles must be respected if human life is to exist. Balancing them is the art of ethics, medicine, and human existence.

1. George Annas, "The Care of Elizabeth Bouvia," *Hastings Center Report* 14(1984): 20.

Suicide: A Rational Choice? 38

When discussing ethical issues surrounding suicide, our main question is not, "Should people who commit suicide be criticized?" Experience and intuition demonstrate that most persons who take their own lives do so because they are emotionally disturbed and act compulsively. Thus their freedom of choice is greatly restricted or nonexistent. Too many of us know dear friends or family members whose suicidal deaths demonstrate the lack of psychological freedom. Indeed, many experts in suicidology today seem to take it for granted that all suicides are compulsive and irrational.[1] Our question in this essay then concerns the contemporary tendency to present suicide as "a rational choice," that is, to present it as the best manner to die in some circumstances.[2]

Discussion

Among the ancient Greeks and Romans, suicide was both condemned and defended, as it also was in Eastern cultures. The Epicureans, who considered pleasure and peace of mind the highest good, argued that it was better to kill oneself than endure life if it had become more painful than pleasurable or peaceful. The Stoics, who believed that rigid self-control was the highest good, argued that it was permissible to kill oneself if suffering or torture might force one to lose self-control. Dualists taught that the soul, which is the real person, is burdened by the body in this life; hence suicide might be justified as a laying down of this burden. Even today, some believe it ethical to choose suicide for the sake of honor. Recently some Irish and Vietnamese chose suicide by self-starvation and self-immolation to protest injustice and oppression.

The monetheistic religions of Judaism, Christianity, and Islam have always opposed suicide, however, because they regard life as God's gift, which people must use not as owners but as faithful stewards. Consequently, we cannot escape accounting to God for our stewardship of this one life given on earth, nor can we reject the body, which will always be part of us. This view was anticipated by Plato, who argued that suicide is a rejection of our responsibility to self, to the community of which one is a part, and to God who gave life. In a different way, another philosopher, Emmanual Kant, argued that suicide is the greatest of crimes because it is a person's rejection of morality itself, since a human being must be his or her own moral lawgiver. Committing suicide means treating oneself as a thing (means) rather than as a person (an end in oneself). In sum, in theological and philosophical reasoning, suicide has been considered for centuries as an unethical act, even though responsibility was seldom imputed to the unfortunate persons who performed the action.

Discussion

Today, however, this classic stand is being called into question. In the United States and England, societies exist that promote suicide as an ethical action, a "rational" alternative to life, especially if a person is beset by depression, loneliness, severe infirmity, or serious suffering. Usually the reasons put forward for approving suicide as an ethical choice are that people should have the right to be autonomous, and to control their own destiny or that people should not have to suffer pain, loneliness, or degradation at the time of death. Although these are professed reasons for the modern reexamination of the traditional stance, a noted psychiatrist and suicidologist, David Peretz, sees a more subtle cause for this change of thought:

> Under the unprecedented stress of recent decades denial mechanisms are breaking down and we have become increasingly vulnerable to the threats of intensely painful feelings of anxiety, fear, panic, rage, guilt, shame, grief, longing and helplessness. In order to avoid being overwhelmed, we seek new ways to

> adapt. . . I believe that the growing
> concern with a good death, death
> with dignity and the right to die
> reflect this search. . . If our deepest
> known fear is of being destroyed, and
> we cannot deal with that fear, we take
> refuge in planning death and rational
> suicide. We find comfort in the
> illusion, "It will not be done to
> me. . . I will do it myself.[3]

Peretz feels this is a dangerous motivation because it fosters the harmful illusion of personal omnipotence.

Two other unrealistic and therefore unethical elements are involved in rational suicide. First, the call for rational suicide is based on the notion that personal autonomy or independence is the goal of human life. Rational suicide says: If one cannot be autonomous or independent, then life is not worth living. This is simply one more expression of radical individualism, a philosophy that weakens human community and places little value on social justice. Both experience and wisdom demonstrate, however, that interdependence, not independence, is the goal of human life. To admit that one is weak and needs help is not a denial or a perversion of one's humanity. Rather, accepting help is a means to fulfill one's humanity. The weak and suffering offer an opportunity to others to fulfill their humanity by responding with care and kindness. The perfectly autonomous person would not need other people; can one imagine a more boring and self-centered individual?

A second unethical element in rational suicide is that it mythologizes the act of self-destruction. To mythologize something is to give it powers it does not possess. Rational suicide presents self-destruction as a problem-free solution to the very serious human problems of physical suffering, loneliness, severe depression, or infirm old age. But we do not eliminate human problems by eliminating human beings. Rather, we eliminate or alleviate human problems through compassion, care, and loving concern. The problems that rational suicide would pretend to eliminate are often problems with which individuals learn to live through the help of caring relatives or friends.

Conclusion

The present-day emphasis on the right to die and death with dignity may blind us to the right to life of the weak, infirm, and aged. The cost of combating the human problems of loneliness, infirmity, and depression is not self-destruction; rather, it is the development of a compassionate, caring, and generous community. Although not simple, this is a development rather than a perversion of our humanity.

1. D. Novak, *Suicide Morality* (New York: Scholars Press, 1971).
2. M. Battin and D. Mayo, eds., *Suicide: The Philosophical Issues* (New York: St. Martin's Press, 1980).
3. D. Peretz, "The Illusion of Rational Suicide," *Hastings Center Report* 11(1981): 40-42.

"Only God Can Heal
My Daughter"

Twelve-year-old Pamela Hamilton broke her leg.[1] When treating her broken leg, her physician discovered a cancerous tumor, which was diagnosed as Ewing's sarcoma. Larry Hamilton, Pamela's father and pastor at the Church of God of the Union Assembly, La Follette, TN, and her mother, Deborah, refused treatment of Pamela's cancer because taking medicine is against their religion. "Only God can heal my daughter," declared her father; "She has the faith to recover; it will be God's will if she does not." Having been notified of Pamela's condition, the Tennessee Department of Social Service petitioned the courts for custody of Pamela on the grounds that her life was endangered because of her parents' religious beliefs. By the time the courts of Tennessee granted the transfer of custody, two months had elapsed. The attending physician stated that she had only a fifty percent chance of survival because of the "red hot and angry tumor which now has spread through her thigh and up to the hip joint." Even though her life was endangered, Pamela agreed with her parent's decision and declared, "I do not want radiation and chemotherapy because I do not want my hair to fall out or to be sick."

Principles

When considering the relationship between parents and children from the Judeo-Christian ethical perspective, two interrelated assumptions are paramount. First, the family unit must be fostered and protected because it is the fundamental element on which society and culture depend for strength and continuity. Second, parents should have care and custody of their children because experience shows that parents love their children and strive to help them become virtuous human beings. Like most ethical assumptions, this latter one yields to contrary evidence. Hence, if parents are abusing their children and endangering their lives, then society intervenes and removes the children from the parents' custody, at least for a time. The right of intervention on behalf of children illustrates another ethical assumption; namely, that parents do not "own" their children. Rather, parents are stewards, caretakers, of their children, enablers who help their children grow in knowledge and virtue. Above all, life and death decisions concerning children are not to be made for the parents' benefit.

Both ethical reasoning and legal precedent give priority to the expression of a person's religious faith. Because religious faith is the most personal, important, and profound act of conscience, its expression should not be limited unless it is manifestly injurious to other people. Hence as long as parents respect the well-being of their children, they have the ethical and legal right to rear and educate their children in the religion of the parents' choice. The right to choose a religion for children, as well as many other rights, gradually wanes as children mature and are able to make competent decisions for themselves. Here, of course, we encounter the crux of the matter: When are children able to make competent decisions for themselves? When do children become young adults? The laws of every country try to solve this question by stating that, for legal purposes, young people become adults at age 17, 18, or 21, depending on the right in question. (Strangely, in most states, young people may marry at an earlier age than they may buy alcoholic beverages.) The laws, however, express only a general norm; it may often happen that a young person is mature enough to make important decisions for himself or herself well before the legal age of maturity. In recognition of this fact, ethicists now suggest that capable children be asked to give their "assent" to surgery or other serious medical treatments, even though the proxy consent of their parents or guardian will suffice for ethical and legal clearance for medical treatment.

Discussion

Cases resembling that of Pamela Hamilton are not unusual. The courts frequently appoint guardians for children whose parents, being Jehovah Witnesses, believe that the Bible prohibits blood transfusions even when death would occur without them. The ethical basis for court action is the assumption that the child's life should not be endangered by the parent's religious beliefs. Even if the child agrees with the parents' belief, the ethical and legal thinking in most of these cases is that the child cannot make a competent decision and, because life is such an important gift, that he or she would choose life if a competent and free decision were possible.

Pamela's situation is different from the usual transfer of custody case for religious reasons. First, she agrees with her parents' decision that she should not receive medicine for treatment of cancer. On the face of it, the parent's statement that "God will cure" is rather unreasonable. Although religious people attribute omnipotence to God and, in that sense, believe that God does cure, they usually do not deny that human beings have a cooperative role to fulfill in effecting a cure. That human beings will one day die is assured, but they have a right and a duty to use positive means such as medicine and surgery to prolong their lives as long as living enables them to pursue the goal of life. But even though the belief of Pamela and her parents seems unreasonable, it is a religious belief and should be honored unless it manifestly harms other people.

This brings us to the second issue that makes Pamela's case somewhat different: there was a threat that she would die within a year even if chemotherapy and radiation were used. The fact that she still survives three years later does not obviate the need for the court to question at the time of the original discussion: What if we take her from her family, give her extensive chemotherapy, and she dies anyway?

In most states, if Pamela were over eighteen and stated that because of her religious beliefs she did not wish to receive medical treatment for her tumor, people might try to persuade her to change her mind, but, in the last analysis, they would be legally and ethically bound to respect her decision. The question that bothers is: Even though she is only twelve years old, did the court make an effort to determine her maturity? No doubt Pamela's faith is strong, but is it due to her parents' influence or to her own free convictions? And did the court consider the gravity of her condition before making its decision?

Conclusion

Given the choice, most people will choose life over death, and legal precedent must be based on what happens most of the time. But legal precedent alone does not guarantee an ethical solution. In order to have an ethical solution, legal precedent must be interpreted in light of the pertinent facts of the case and the ethical assumptions on which the precedent is based. Pamela's case reminds us that religious and family rights are very important and that the courts must consider particular facts and assumptions as well as precedent in order to form ethical decisions.

---

1. Fourteen-year-old Pamela Hamilton died from cancer in 1985. Although Pamela eventually received treatment and her cancer was considered in remission as of September 1984, she was rediagnosed as terminal in 1985. (*American Medical News,* May 20, 1985).

End Stage Renal Disease: 40
An Ethical Evaluation

In 1972 the federal government passed legislation to assume the costs for transplantation and dialysis for anyone with severe renal disease (ESRD). The purpose of this program was to sustain life for those who suffered kidney disease, to make life more beneficial for those suffering from this disease, and, above all, to make this life-saving treatment available to all, no matter what their level of income or place in society.

In 1974, the first year of the program, about 5,000 patients were treated; the cost was $172 million. According to the latest figures, in 1985 the cost for the ESRD program is estimated at $2 billion, and about 60,000 people will be cared for; about 5,000 will receive kidney transplants.[1]

Principles

What are the results of the ESRD program? Surely the lives of many people have been prolonged through transplants and dialysis; family members have benefitted as well. Sustaining life through transplantation or dialysis, however, does not lead to a problem-free existence. Even for those with successful transplantations, debilitating physiological and psychological problems can occur.

But even if dialysis or transplant prolongs life, it does not solve all problems. The type of burden that afflicts those with transplants is summed up in the words of a transplant patient:

> The dramatic character of transplantation diverts attention from social problems inherent in the medical procedures, such as failure of the operation to meet expectations of the patient and family, disruption of family equilibrium, and investment of public funds to meet these costs.

Renal failure and transplantation precipitates a crisis that may be defined differently by the patient and family. The crisis situation may mobilize or it may incapacitate them.[2]

For those who remain on dialysis, the problems seem to be more serious. A recent survey of men and women in several dialysis centers found that among diabetic patients, over fifty percent were not able to care for themselves completely.[3] In contrast, only about twenty percent of nondiabetic patients were judged to be unable to care for themselves completely. Overall, the results of this survey suggest that at least forty percent of dialysis patients have not achieved successful occupational rehabilitation and that at least one of five patients is unable to live an independent existence. The survey indicated that in 1979, forty-four percent of the patients observed were not working, and more than fifty percent were probably too sick to work, irrespective of their level of education and previous employment status. Although hemodialysis alleviates the uremic syndrome and the patient generally feels better, there are diet restrictions, problems with blood pressure, feelings of weakness, impotence, periodical hospitalization, and shunt complications, any of which may prevent participation in daily activities.

Discussion

Even though many people on dialysis lead a debilitated existence, given the main purpose and objectives of the ESRD program, it seems that the program has been an outstanding success because it fulfills the ethical values of medicine and the goals of a compassionate society. The lives of thousands have been prolonged; no question is asked about the income, social standing, or productivity of the people who receive therapy. Moreover, the families of renal dialysis patients are able to share life more abundantly with their loved ones. There are those who believe the ESRD program has been a disaster, however, because it is so expensive and does not totally "cure" people. Usually, when people of this opinion evaluate this

ESRD program they start out by computing the cost and decrying the fact that the cost has escalated considerably over the years. In addition to decrying the cost, subtle hints are given that we are keeping alive the "useless" members of society because we are prolonging life for those who cannot hold a job and are therefore nonproductive.

For example, the aforementioned study suggests "that a much larger number of American dialysis patients are severely debilitated than has been previously anticipated or reported."[4] The implication of this study is that because many people receiving dialysis do not lead "productive lives," the program is flawed. The assumption seems to be that only those who are "productive" are worthwhile. We find this attitude ethically unsound and inhumane as well. We must be very careful about evaluating persons solely on the basis of productivity, else we affirm a materialistic and pragmatic ethic—an ethic that, history demonstrates, eliminates the weak, the infirm, and the socially undesirable under the guise of efficiency, financial need, or social progress.

For many people, the only evaluation of health care programs is a financial evaluation. Let us realize, however, that making or saving money is not the goal of a compassionate society. The gross national product is not the standard of ethical activity. Rather, we should realize that our financial considerations should be at the service of our ethical standards. Our budgets, our financial planning, should be the expression of our ethical philosophy.

Two billion dollars is a large sum, but the overall decision on whether this program is affordable must be worked out with a view to the nation's total assets, the amount of public funds that should be devoted to health care needs, and the priorities that should be developed for public and private health care funds. In other words, we cannot ignore how much our health care programs cost, but we must put the cost in perspective. We can only do this rationally and consistently if we develop national health care priorities for a humane, ethical, and just society. We must realize that we have limited means and plan our life-prolonging programs of the future within those means.

Conclusion

The call for priorities and planning within the national health care program is nothing new. Fifteen years ago, when Medicare was introduced, such a statement of priorities was called for. To date, no consensus in regard to priorities has been developed, which is one reason why an adversarial relationship has developed between the federal government and health care professionals.

1. *AHA Washington Memo*, 3/1/85; p. 8.
2. Mark Reinsberg and Patricia C. Laney, "Surviving," *Nursing '76*, (April 1976): 47-49.
3. R. A. Gutman, et al., "Physical Activity and Employment Status of Patients on Maintenance Dialysis," *New England Journal of Medicine* 304(1981): 309-313.
4. Gutman, 313.

Physicians and Stress   41
in the Twenty-first Century

Another scholarly article has appeared in a national medical journal depicting the stresses that occur in physicians' life and the inadequate manner in which many physicians cope with stress. The author, Jack McCue, MD, believes that:

> The stresses in medical practice result from one or more of the following situations peculiar to medicine: working with intensely emotional aspects of life governed by strong cultural code for behavior, e.g., suffering, fear, sexuality and death; inadequate training for fundamental professional tasks, e.g., handling "problem" patients; and demands from society or patients that cannot be reasonably met, e.g., the need for certainty when current medical knowledge allows only approximation.[1]

Principles

After analyzing these stress factors, Dr. McCue offers a resume of the effects of stress on physicians:

> It is certain that physicians who harm themselves also directly or indirectly harm their patients. Ample evidence indicates that physician impairment is common. The suicide rate of physicians is two to three times that of the general population. Alcoholism is at least as prevalent among physicians as in the general

population, and underreporting of physician-alcoholics is likely. Drug addiction may be 30-100 times more common among physicians than in the general population, a controlled study shows that heavy drug use, including use of alcohol, was 1.6 times more frequent among doctors than in a comparable group of non-physicians. Physicians are likely to have 10 or more visits to a psychiatrist than are controls.[2]*

Dr. McCue's article is remarkable, but not because it contains new information concerning physician impairment, nor because it offers any new or different solutions. Several other articles have appeared in the last few years that present similar statistics and scenarios and that offer similar solutions. All emphasize two things: (1) the problems that become acute in later life for physicians are seminally present in medical school and residency programs; and (2) very little is being done in medical schools and residency programs to help physicians prepare competently for the stresses they will encounter throughout their practice. Hence, Dr. McCue's article is remarkable because in spite of his observations and similar other articles indicating serious problems, to date little has been done in medical schools to prepare future physicians for personal and social problems.

Discussion

How is stress in physicians' lives related to ethics? Ethics is concerned not only with solving problems, but, more

---

*Although suicide, alcoholism, and drug addiction indicate a poor reaction to stress, visits to a psychiatrist should not be used as an indicator of stress. We all encounter stress; impairment occurs because one copes poorly with it. Seeking the help of a psychiatrist, however, can be a very effective way to cope with stress.

important, with ordering life. Thus the ethical physician would seek to avoid impairment rather than be involved in the issues that surround incipient or developing impairment. How would he or she seek to avoid ineffective coping with inevitable stresses? Briefly, the person would spend time pondering three things: first, what objectives should I have and which are more important; second, what is my motivation for being a physician; third, what are my assets and limitations. To discern these things, any person needs the help of others, and the responses will change over time; hence there must be periodic reflection on these questions. If any person does not engage in such self-renewal, he or she will get in a rut, find life very frustrating, and eventually suffer burnout.

What has been said about the ethical individual who wishes to integrate his or her life and cope with the stress that each person must expect to encounter is true also of institutions. That is, the persons who make up any institution must come together periodically and reflect on their objectives, motivations, strengths, and weaknesses. Otherwise, the institution will get in a rut and suffer burnout. How often do medical schools— administration, faculty, and students—engage in such reflection? One of the great breakthroughs in the history of medical education occurred when the *Flexner Report* was written and implemented in the early 20th century. Is it time for another effort to assess medical education in view of the changing times, the intense stresses that occur, and patients' needs to be cared for by competent physicians? (Since this article was written the Association of American Medical Colleges produced a report on *The General Professional Education of Physicians* (GPEP Report, 1984).[3] While the GPEP Report offers some beneficial ideas for change in medical education, it is too soon to determine whether the ideas will be implemented.)

Conclusion

Several beneficial changes have occurred in the last few years in curriculum, student counseling services, examination schedules, and class hours in medical schools, but are these changes sufficient to effect the type of renewal needed to prepare competent physicians for the 21st century? Such physicians must not only be prepared to learn and apply the new technology and scientific information in accord with the ethical ideals of their profession, but they must also be able to cope with the increased stress that will occur in their lives.

1. "The Effects of Stress on Physicians and Their Medical Practice," *New England Journal of Medicine*, 306(2/25/82): 458-468.
2. "Effects of Stress," 460.
3. *The General Professional Education of Physicians*, Washington, DC: Association of American Medical Colleges, 1984.

The Human Factor   42
in Medical Error

In 1981 two articles evaluating the performance of
health care professionals appeared in the *New England
Journal of Medicine*. One article reported "a one year
prospective survey to identify adverse outcomes due to error
during care in the field of general surgery."[1] The other studied
"iatrogenic illnesses on a general medical service at a
university hospital."[2] Because the topic of error is significant
for everyone associated with health care, especially patients,
these articles deserve consideration from an ethical point of
view. The article evaluating error in patient care in general
surgery reported that the approximate incidence of
complicated cases amounted to about one percent. Fifty-six
important errors in all occurred; in eleven cases the patients
died, with surgical mistakes a contributing factor. The origins
of error were identified as misplaced optimism, unwarranted
urgency, urge for perfection, and vogue therapy. "The
predominant example of fallibility appears to have been
insufficient restraint and deliberation. Excessive haste,
impatience, overconfidence and inadequate peer group
consultation were important influences in this regard." All the
errors seem to be due to error of judgment rather than error of
negligence, however.

The second article, concerned with medical service,
defined iatrogenic illness as "any illness that resulted from a
diagnostic procedure or from any form of therapy, or harmful
occurrences that were not natural consequences of a patient's
disease." This study reported on 815 patients; of these, 290 (36
percent) had one or more iatrogenic illnesses, with a total of
497 such occurrences. A total of 76 patients (9 percent of all
those admitted) had major complications. In 15 cases, the
iatrogenic illness was believed to have contributed to the
patient's death. The three causes of most iatrogenic events
were drugs, cardiac catherizations, and falls. Of all patients
with complications, 53 percent had at least one problem
related to drug exposure.

Discussion

The hospital trustees, administrators, and medical personnel responsible for these studies are to be commended for the thorough evaluation of their work. Thorough evaluation of one's efforts in order to improve effectiveness is an ethical responsibility, especially when the effort in question is concerned with important human values, such as health and life. Through surveys of this nature, even though they may be painful, health care professionals should be able to determine the prevalence of avoidable errors and establish surveillance and educational procedures that will minimize them. Something similar to these studies should be instituted in each reputable health care facility so that greater proficiency and accountability result.

Two sources of error and iatrogenic illness exist, namely, mistaken judgment and negligence. In every way possible, negligence must be guarded against by physicians and other health care professionals. Methods and procedures must be instituted to control and, if possible, eliminate negligence. These studies show, however, that even when negligence is minimized or eliminated, the potential for error and complication still remains through mistaken judgment. Thus the fact that medicine is not an exact science is once again demonstrated vividly. In both surgery and medicine, many things, especially patients' reactions to particular drugs or procedures, cannot be predicted in advance. Although good physicians are careful, if they were to act only when they were absolutely certain, they would not act very often. This is the nature of the service they offer. Most health care workers realize the potential fallibility of their judgments, but the general public perhaps does not. Many patients have unrealistic expectations of health care professionals; often they are frustrated and angry when these expectations are not fulfilled. Thus better relationships between health care professionals and patients would exist if the nature of medicine were clearly understood by all concerned.

As the authors of the medical study indicate, the risk incurred during hospitalization is not trivial. Thus serious considerations should be given to new methods of monitoring untoward occurrences in hospitalized patients, especially those caused by drugs. Some might respond that most hospitals already have committees that should attend to the incidence of iatrogenic complications. Are the processes most hospitals use to evaluate quality care as thorough as those indicated in the aforementioned articles? Moreover, are such studies ever made public? A recognized expert in hospital administration states that few hospitals would have good enough records to allow quality assurance studies of this nature. Although the Joint Committee on Accreditation (JCAH) does make some effort to have hospitals evaluate their services, the methods used depend on the local health care facility. Thus the objectivity and openness needed to produce effective quality care studies is not often present. In a profession, in order to ensure competent service and personal satisfaction, peer evaluation and peer discipline are needed. Are these two characteristics fully operative at present in the health care profession?

The surgical study emphasizes that complications arising from physicians' errors contribute to the high cost of medical care. No one can deny that complications in surgery and medicine will increase the cost of health care, but is this the major reason why health care professionals should be concerned about preventing surgical errors and iatrogenic illness? Should not they be more concerned about the effect these errors and complications have on the patient, the physician, and other health care professionals? Not one word is offered in the articles about patient suffering or family sorrow due to errors by physicians or hospital personnel, nor is there any mention of the anguish, sorrow, and self-doubt in health care workers. There is a degrading and dangerous tendency— degrading to the health care professional and dangerous to the patient—to make cost and economics the principal standard by which medicine and health care are evaluated. This tendency is most obvious when people speak about the "health care *industry*." Health care is not an industry; it is a profession. As such, its first standard of evaluation for its efforts is patient well-being and human welfare. Although monetary factors must be considered, they should not dominate or control the evaluation of health care.

1. N. P. Couch, et al., "The High Cost of Low-Frequency Events," *New England Journal of Medicine* 304(1981): 634-637.
2. Knight Steel, MD, et al., "Iatrogenic Illness on a General Medical Service at a University Hospital," *New England Journal of Medicine*, 304(1981): 638-641.

The Infant Doe Case   43

In 1982, in Indiana, a newborn boy with Down's syndrome and esophageal atresia died because care was withheld. Physicians advising the parents said they had an ethical right to choose surgery to correct the digestive defect or to choose to do nothing. The parents chose to withhold all food and drink from the baby, thus ensuring that he would die. The hospital asked for a legal ruling, and two Bloomington, IN, judges upheld the parents' right to withhold care and surgical treatment. The county prosecutor became interested in the case, asking the Indiana Supreme Court to override the judges' decision. The Court refused, by a 3-1 vote, thus supporting the parents' right to withhold treatment.[1]

Briefly, those are the facts of the "Infant Doe case." A sustained cry of outrage and an equally vociferous defense of the action were heard in response to the case. Personally, we think it a good sign when people are interested enough to get excited. People should get excited about life and death decisions; otherwise, where is our compassion and mercy? But "getting excited" is not a sufficient response to a serious ethical issue. Unless our emotional response is founded on ethical principles, it is liable to do more harm than good. In this essay, then, we would like to consider the Infant Doe case from an ethical perspective. Before doing so, however, some of the misrepresentations from press and public resulting from emotional response are listed: (1) the impression was given that every infant, no matter what the medical difficulties, should be kept alive as long as possible; (2) the lawyer sought to justify the parents' ethical decision by saying "it was a difficult case;" (3) withholding food and water was described as "letting nature take its course;" (4) the terms *ordinary means* and *extraordinary means* were used constantly and confusedly with no understanding of their meanings; and (5) lawyers and editorial writers were informing us "authoritatively" about medical decisions.

Principles

    The ethics of medicine mandate that life be prolonged as long as the person whose life is in the balance can strive for the purpose of life. The assumption of medicine, not unlike the assumption in religious thought, is that life is good and should be prolonged so that people may enjoy it and fulfill its meaning. If disease or illness seems to threaten life, the question is asked, Should life be prolonged? The response to this question would be yes, unless it is found that one will not be able to strive for the purpose of life if life is prolonged. We find the possibility of one's striving for the purpose of life by asking two questions; if either question is answered yes, then it is permissible to allow the person to die because striving for the purpose of life is no longer possible. The first question is: Will the therapy be useless? The second question is: Will prolonging life cause a grave burden for the person whose life is threatened (i.e., make it very difficult for the person to strive for the goal of life)? Because of our respect for persons and their right to life, the decision whether to prolong life usually should be made by the person whose life is endangered. If this person is unable to decide, the family becomes involved; their proxy decision is respected unless it seems detrimental to the patient's best interests. In this latter case, the court may be asked to intervene. In all situations, the physician offers advice and counsel but does not have the right to make the final decision.

Discussion

    Let us apply this reasoning to the case of Infant Doe. Would surgery for esophageal atresia be useless? For surgery to be useless, it means that it will not prolong life for any significant time in regard to achieving the purpose of life. Could Infant Doe's life have been prolonged for a significant time if the surgery for esophageal atresia were performed? We cannot answer that question accurately because we do not have the necessary medical information. We have tried to obtain this information, but the records of the case have been sealed by order of the Supreme Court of Indiana. If esophageal atresia were the only life-threatening cause, then surgery should have been performed, because all indications are that this surgery usually prolongs life for a significant time. Serious heart condition, however, is often present in children with Down's syndrome and esophageal atresia. If this heart condition were not curable through surgery, then the answer to the question of whether surgery would be useless might be yes. Although we cannot answer this question adequately because of the lack of information, we can say that if the only birth anomaly were esophageal atresia, surgery should most likely have been performed. A good norm in such cases is: Surgery should not be withheld simply because a person has Down's syndrome.

Could living with Down's syndrome be considered a grave burden insofar as attaining the purpose of life is concerned? People with Down's syndrome are capable of loving relationships and other actions associated with the purpose of life. Hence it would be very difficult to maintain that the malady of Down's syndrome is in itself a grave burden. Perhaps rearing a child with Down's syndrome would be a grave burden for some parents, but the proxy decision must be directed toward the patient's, not the parents' or society's benefit. Depending on the extent of the burden, society should help the family rear children. Thus life for Infant Doe could not be considered a grave burden.

To complete this brief analysis, two more thoughts should be expressed. First, in ethics, the term *ordinary means* implies that some medicine or therapy is necessary; that is, it would be unethical or immoral to withhold it. The term *extraordinary means* implies that the same medicine or therapy is optional; it may be used, but need not be. Determining whether some particular means to prolong life is necessary or optional occurs after the decision on whether to prolong life has been made. When prolonging life is the ethical responsibility, then the means to that end are called "ordinary" (e.g., a respirator); when a person will be allowed to die, the same identical means are declared "extraordinary." Second, because medicine is concerned with caring as well as curing, water and food should be offered to a dying person if they are means of comfort (Conroy case p. 216-219). Even if medical reasons had indicated that treatment of Infant Doe was useless, he should have been given water through intravenous feeding and other therapy to reduce or relieve pain.

Questions concerning the treatment of dying people will confront us dramatically in the coming years. We must strive for ethical consensus, or the issue will divide our society. Fortunately, the President's Commission for the Study of Ethical Problems in Medicine provided a forum for discussion. This commission has done some worthwhile studies and has considered the question of allowing persons to die. With the results of this study, let us, when confronting serious ethical issues, seek to analyze ethically before allowing our emotions to dictate our response.

---

1. Martin Gerry, "The Civil Rights of Handicapped Infants," *Issues in Law and Medicine*, 1(July 1985): 5.

Federal regulations have been published to guide decision making for impaired newborns, requiring that all such children receive medical attention that would be to their benefit and making it a violation of civil rights legislation if such therapy is withheld from them because they are handicapped.[1] This new ruling, referred to as the Baby Doe regulations, is the result of the controversy surrounding the Down's syndrome child born in 1982, in Bloomington, IN, who was refused surgery for esophageal atresia. There are other similar cases; among them Baby Ashley, an anencephalic child abandoned in Idaho, and Baby Jane Doe, who suffers from an improperly fused spine and other neurological defects. The treatment of these children raises ethical, social, and medical questions. Technology makes it possible to save some of these children who, fifteen years ago, would have died shortly after birth. Underneath the debate about which of these children should be saved are two questions: Is it better for some of these children to die rather than live? What should we do with these children and who should decide? These questions raise serious issues about the method of medical decision making.

Principles

Central to the medical decision to treat or not to treat a child is the issue of whether the treatment is of benefit to the

*Three sets of federal regulations were published regarding medical treatment of impaired newborn infants. In the following three essays, we offer an ethical evaluation of these regulations written at the time the regulations were issued. At present only the regulations issued on April 15, 1985 are operative because the first two sets of regulations were declared unconstitutional by federal district courts. However, should the Supreme Court determine that the original regulations were incorrectly declared unconstitutional, then the original regulations would be reinstated.

child. Benefit presumes underlying principles, specifically that one does not lose one's right to life by virtue of having a birth defect or because one will be mentally impaired. Life does not have to be perfect in order to be valued. On the other hand, life is not valued simply because mere physiological function is maintained in a technological fashion. Other significant values exist beyond mere physical function. The quality of the child's life is important, too, and though it is a difficult factor to judge, it must be considered in life-prolonging decisions.

The President's Commission for the Study of Ethical Problems in Medicine lists three categories of infants to help simplify the decision-making process in regard to prolonging life.[2] In the first category are those infants for whom treatment is beneficial; the second are those for whom treatment is futile; and in the third are those for whom treatment is uncertain.

The first category includes defective children who may benefit from the correction of some anomaly or secondary problem even when other primary anomalies are not correctable. This occurred in the Indiana Baby Doe case. The Down's syndrome child with esophageal atresia and no other defects will benefit from the surgical procedure, allowing the child to receive and perhaps give love, live in a family, and, perhaps, with luck, be educable. What is not considered in the benefit analysis is the fact that the child has and will forever have a mental impairment. The child does not lose a right to life and treatment simply because of this chromosomal anomaly.

The second category includes children for whom the most aggressive help is useless. The child with an hypo-plastic heart serves as an example. Regardless of how aggressive the treatment is, the child will die soon. Little can be done to correct the incomplete development of the child's heart. Little can be offered. The child does not benefit, because all that is offered is the prolongation of physiological existence and the process of dying. When the family and physicians reach an agreement to withdraw treatment, there is no ethical problem.

The third category contains the greater number of children and placement in this group leads to difficult ethical decisions. This group generally contains children with multiple anomalies requiring serious attention. The outlook for this group can be complicated by the fact that therapy itself may aggravate or contribute to still further difficulties. The most aggressive treatment of these children may prolong life for a short time. The difficulty is that these children are not born dying; their prognosis is uncertain. They may have a few months or years of life and may be able to go home, but none of that will be possible without some immediate medical attention. More than the above two categories, this category raises serious questions about the method by which medical decisions are made.

Discussion

Ethical consideration in these cases is generally a reflection on whether good medicine is practiced, the patient's rights and dignity are respected, and the decision-making process is just. The following points must be considered: First, in almost all cases the best decisions are those made in conjunction with the physician, medical staff, and family. Parents play a crucial role. This may be complicated by the shock of a defective newborn, a mother recuperating in another hospital, and a father with other familial responsibilities. Regardless of these difficulties, parents should not be excluded from ethical decisions, unless their decision clearly disrespects the child's life. In addition, decision making is important for their own health, especially where grieving, understanding the child's congenital problems, and resolving possible guilt feelings or arrangements to care for the child and other options are concerned.

Second, time is of the essence for the medical team. Seldom is a child born whose medical complications are immediately obvious at birth. Although birth weight and initial extrauterine signs may be helpful, they are frequently not decisive. Accurate assessment of the child's mental and physical condition takes time. In such cases, aggressive therapy may be called for until it becomes medically clear the child is dying or that continued aggressive therapy is no longer in the child's best interest.

Third, the future of an impaired child may depend in part on the parents' ability to adjust to the reality of the child, counsel with their religious leaders, seek additional information from parents of similarly affected children, and examine the alternatives available to them. Again, time is necessary.

Conclusion

Clearly, not all impaired newborns can be saved, and at times they must be allowed to die. These children raise uncomfortable questions that we must address. What should society do in assisting these children and their families? What role does the handicapped child play in our society? Why do we have children, and what should we do when we have impaired children? Why are perfect children the only acceptable ones? Why do parents feel guilty when they have a impaired child? Are children labeled "retarded" and deemed less valuable only because they cannot perform with the finely honed cognitive skills? Why do we spend almost two billion dollars a year in neonatal intensive care units if we do not want to spend money caring for the least advantaged among us? The questions are unsettling. They will not go away. They will not be solved by new federal regulations. Each impaired child born in our society will cause us to ask the questions anew.

1. *Federal Register* 47, 26027(1982), May 18.
2. President's Commission for the Study of Ethical Problems in Medicine and Biomedical and Behavioral Research, *Deciding to Forego Life-Sustaining Treatment,* (Washington, DC: U. S. Government Printing Office, 1983), p. 214.

In the spring of 1982 in Indiana, a boy born with Down's syndrome and esophageal atresia died because food and water were withheld with approval of the local court. (See the preceding essay.) The infant became known as Baby Doe, and, in response to the case, the Department of Health and Human Services has issued regulations seeking to protect the lives of handicapped infants under the Civil Rights Act. The first set of regulations were declared unconstitutional primarily because time was not allowed for comments. The second regulations are the subject of this essay.[1] Calling for infant care review committees (ICRCs) to assist in ethical decision making and the posting of signs containing relevant telephone numbers where violations for withholding care from infants on the basis of handicaps may be reported, the regulations significantly modify current procedures.

Principles

The apparent assumptions of the document are even more significant than the regulations. They are:

1. Common standards or principles for ethical action can be developed for our pluralistic society. Ethics, then, is not based on intuition or on an emotional response to conflict; rather, it is based on a reasoned and systematic evaluation of human need. A just and compassionate application of the standards in question depends on an ability to understand the grounding of the principles and an accurate knowledge of the facts of the particular case. This is a long overdue realization.

2. For centuries, society has respected the responsibility of parents, with the advice of physicians, to decide within reasonable limits the proper treatment for their infants suffering from severe birth defects. Now other people serving on ICRCs have the right to advise parents, and hospitals in some cases must put the case before the court. This is a radical change; is it needed? The federal government, supported by several disability organizations, such as the

Down's Syndrome Congress and the Spina Bifida Association, and citing several articles and surveys, assumes that physicians have abused their power.

Ethically speaking, the significant parts of the document are the sections on "Principles for Treatment of Disabled Infants" and "Guidelines for Applicability." The main statements are as follows:

a. Health care providers may not, solely on the basis of present or anticipated physical or mental impairments of an infant, withhold treatment or nourishment from the infant who in spite of such impairment will medically benefit from the treatment or nourishment.

b. Consideration such as anticipated or actual limited potential of an individual and present or future lack of available community resources are irrelevant and must not determine the decisions concerning medical care.

c. This standard is very strict and it excludes consideration of the negative effects of an impaired child's life on other persons, including parents, siblings and society.[2]

Discussion

The key concept in the document is that treatment must be given if it is "medically beneficial." What does this mean? Judging from the examples and content of the document, the document assumes treatment should be judged medically beneficial if it will prolong life for a significant time. Only when "medical care is futile and only prolongs the act of dying" may treatment be withheld; "a presumption always should be in favor of treatment" if doubt exists on the value of treatment (p. 1652).

Thus the judgment on "medically beneficial" seems to consider only one human function, the physiological. Any disability, no matter how severe, in the psychological, the social, and the cognitive-affective functions may not be the basis for withholding treatment. Moreover, life must be prolonged no matter what the cost to community or family. We submit that this method of ethical decision making is erroneous as well as contrary to the Catholic tradition in medical ethics. We refer to the Catholic tradition not because it is normative for our society, but because it represents an acknowledged pro-life position.[3] The federal norms are more strict and rigid than the Catholic tradition.

To understand our position, recall that the Catholic tradition does not make physiological existence an end in itself. We live in order to fulfill the goal of life. No matter how we define the goal of life, e.g., happiness, serving our neighbor, serving God, doing God's will, reaching our potential, we must have, *at least potentially* some degree of cognitive-affective function. Thus functions over and above the physiological are considered when making decisions about care for self or others. When making judgments about whether to prolong the life of older people, we consider these functions frequently. When an older person is in an irreversible coma, thus lacking potential for cognitive-affective, social, and psychological function, we determine that life-support systems may be removed, even though physiological function could be prolonged.

Another criterion of Judeo-Christian ethics for prolonging life in the presence of pathological conditions is whether the person would find life a grave burden. Would prolonging life involve excruciating pain; would surgeries deplete financial resources; would continued care present a continuing grave burden on the rest of the family? If so, one may forego life-prolonging treatment and request to be allowed to die.

When making a proxy decision for medical care of another, whether that person be elderly and comatose or a mere infant struggling for life, the same ethical principles should be used. The proxy puts himself or herself in the patient's place and asks, "What is beneficial for me as a total human person?" Does any responsible and reasonable person determine what is beneficial for himself or herself by abstracting from family and society? We think not. None of us has the right to burden excessively the people with whom we live. True, infants' chances of survival are difficult to pinpoint, so we must give them the benefit of the doubt; however, the decision must take into account more than capacity to prolong physiological existence.

Clearly, a mistake was made in the Indiana Baby Doe case, but let us not compound it. Handicapped infants must be protected because life is a great gift. Review committees could help parents, physicians, and hospital administrators make compassionate and ethical decisions. But all concerned must make decisions on sound ethical principles. We are open to correction, but it seems that the federal government has not provided the proper principles and guidelines for the task.

---

1. "Principles for Treatment of Disabled Infants," 45 CFR, Part 84, January 12, 1984. These regulations were declared unconstitutional by a Federal Court, but the decision is being appealed to the Supreme Court. In the meantime, the Department of Health & Human Service has issued new regulations (See p. 177).
2. "Principles for Treatment," p. 1652-1653.
3. "On Euthanasia," Congregation of Doctrine of the Faith, 6/26/80; cf. Pius XII, "Prolonging Life," 11/24/57.

On April 15, 1985, the latest Baby Doe regulations were published in the *Federal Register*.[1] These rules are not attachments to the antidiscrimination rules, as were the earlier ones, but are related to the Child Abuse Prevention and Treatment Act as amended by Congress in 1984. Principally, the final ruling requires that the Child Protection Agency (CPS) of each state establish and maintain a method of receiving complaints about child abuse when medical neglect is concerned and establish contacts with individual hospitals in order to facilitate, by whatever appropriate means necessary, the proper medical treatment of all medically neglected children.

Hospitals are required by the legislation to provide the name, title, and telephone number of the contact person(s) of their institution to the CPS agencies so that proper contact can be made when necessary. In addition, the hospitals should provide the necessary information so that all people (and not just the nurses and physicians) can make known suspected cases of child abuse involving medical neglect. It is encouraged, although not mandated, that institutions establish infant care review committees (ICRCs), which would be responsible for reviewing cases of the withdrawal and withholding of medical care from infants, promoting education about these matters in the institution, and developing appropriate policy when necessary (14893-14901).

The heart of the rules is the same as the previous Baby Doe regulations. No child for whom any treatment is beneficial should have medical treatment withheld or withdrawn. The regulations employ various principles in articulating this position.

Principles

The most fundamental principle used in the regulations requires normal or reasonable medical judgment to be made, where reasonable medical judgment is defined as that which a reasonably prudent physician would make knowing the case and the available options (14888). Unlike previous legislation, the current regulations offer no suggestions about appropriate therapies for particular diseases.

Second, the regulations require that appropriate nutrition, hydration, and medication always be given (14878). When discussing the types of cases in which treatment may not be medically indicated, the regulations are very clear that this does not include appropriate nutrition, hydration, and medication. In the appendix to the rule, some light is shed on the fact that medication should be understood in light of the infant's need for proper palliation (14892). Later in the appendix it is stated that the word *appropriate* is clear and the rule intends in an "unequivocal" fashion that no child be denied appropriate nutrition, hydration, and medication.

Third, the future quality of the infant's life is not a concern in making these decisions. As such, the rule excludes the use of any subjective factors in decision making and discounts future possibilities or probabilities from medical decision making. This attempts to guarantee the "sacredness of life" of each child.

Last, to implement these rules, the regulations suggest the establishment of an ICRC in each institution to educate, consult, and decide on certain policies. Although no particular structure is mandated, the regulations offer a detailed sketch of one possible committee.

Discussion

The provision of adequate medical care is a goal for all infants regardless of their medical status. Whether adequate medical care, as envisioned by the Department of Health and Human Services and the congressional legislation on which these rules are based, will be realized is a question as yet unanswered.

The first principle (reasonable medical judgment by a prudent physician) presumably requires a consensual decision-making process with the parents of the child in question and reflects the very basis of medicine and medical ethics.

Medicine is not a strict science. It uses science in trying to make decisions that benefit patients. There must be a great deal of latitude in the decision-making process because no illness is the same in two different patients. Reasonable medical judgment is an appropriate ethical principle. The difficulty in this part of the legislation is the presence of a "clearinghouse" that will provide "expert medical advice and information" (14887). Diseases cannot be categorized so easily. In addition, especially for affected neonates, the various complications are such that the treatment for a particular child may be unique. Those who insist on the computer's information as vital to the appropriateness of the medical decision may undermine the very possibility of good medical practice.

The second principle (appropriate nutrition, hydration, and medication) poses difficulties. There is a moral demand to feed people, especially when the lack of food may cause pain. If and when that moral demand is no longer present, however, is an issue confronting medical ethics today. One cannot accept starving someone to death simply because it is more economical or convenient or because someone is not wanted. Clearly, these actions are unethical. There are times, however, when a child is unable to eat (because of an irreversible coma, for instance). Forced feeding could be instituted, but the question is, Why?

It may be that there is great emotional meaning to feeding such a child. If so, perhaps this can be accepted as a kind gesture by society. One should not confuse this pressing emotional need with an ethical obligation, however. The two are not always the same. Appropriate nutrition and hydration and medication can be ethical obligations if one realizes that appropriate nutrition in some cases can mean no forced feedings, hydration, or medicine. Like other therapies, food, water, and medication are related to the meaning and purpose of life. More clarity and ethical reflection are needed; there is more ambiguity than clarity in this principle.

Third, the issue of quality of life needs attention. If by quality of life one means that no arbitrary decision should be made about the value of a person's life, then indeed quality of life decisions are inappropriate—not only for infants but for every patient. If, however, what is implied by quality of life is a careful statement about the burdens borne by the child, or the suffering that will be entailed in the child's life, then quality issues pose a central problem. The regulations point to the uselessness of treatment as a criterion by which one decides in certain cases not to continue certain types of treatment. The regulations do not recognize, however, that ethically two standards or criteria have been used in determining when it is time to allow a person to die. The first is the uselessness of the medical therapy, but the second is burden to the patient. Assessing burden is a difficult task. Ultimately, it must be guided by an attempt to realize the child's best interest.

The future quality of the child's life, contrary to the regulations, is a primary concern. The ability of the child to be free of pain, free of neonatal intensive care units, able, however minimally, to experience aspects of life other than medical care, are significant. If one does not consider the future quality of the child's life, one may focus on the physical life of the child and prolong the child's dying rather than the child's living.

Finally, an ICRC or any other appropriate committee may help to ensure a good decision if it attends to educational needs and proper policy development. Structures that allow committees to veto physician-parent decisions or act as medical decision makers may create barriers to sound medical decision making.

The issue of federal regulations governing decisions in neonatal intensive care units is not over. However, one thing is clear, sound medicine and consensual decision making between parents and providers is more likely to ensure good decisions than are federal regulations.

Footnote

1. *Federal Register* (Washington, DC: U.S. Government Printing Office, April 15, 1985).

Perhaps a few people living on the back of the moon have not heard of Baby Fae, but most of us are familiar with her struggle for life as the first infant to receive a transplant of a baboon heart. Although she lived just short of three weeks with the transplant, the medical treatment she received spawned a host of ethical questions that live after her. We shall consider some of these questions in this essay.

Principles

When doing research involving human subjects, most physicians and scientists in the United States follow regulations for ethical research published by agencies of the federal government. Indeed, if the research in question is funded by the federal government, following the federal regulations is mandatory. Evaluating human research protocols to ensure conformity with federal regulations is the responsibility of the institutional review board (IRB). An IRB, required at every research institution, is mainly concerned with protecting the human subjects involved in research projects, but has some concern with the scientific validity of the project as well. At some schools, Saint Louis University for example, all research projects involving human subjects must be approved by the IRB, not only those funded by the federal government.

The federal regulations for research involving children envision two types of research: that which "holds out prospects of direct benefit for the individual subject" and that which "does not hold out the prospect of direct benefit for the individual subject."[1] In this latter type of research there may be a benefit resulting from the study, such as new scientific knowledge, that would benefit other children, but there is no direct benefit for the child or children involved in the research project. Concerning the first type of research, which involves therapeutic treatment for the child or children in question, the regulations for ethical research are similar to those regulating research on adult human subjects. Hence consent must be received (in this case proxy consent, because the child cannot give informed consent) and the risk of harm envisioned must be justified by the anticipated benefit.

In regard to the research on children who do not benefit directly, however, the regulations are more involved.

First, a distinction is made between "minimal risk of harm" to the subject and "more than minimal risk of harm." *Minimal risk* is equivalent to "physical and psychological harm that is normally encountered in the daily lives or in the routine medical or psychological examination of healthy children." Research that involves *"more than* minimal risk" may be approved by the IRB if there is "only a *minor increase* over minimal risk" and other requirements are met. If the IRB finds that the research involves a *major increase* over minimal risk, "the IRB can refer the project to the Department of Health and Human Services for study by a panel of experts," provided the IRB also "finds that the research presents a reasonable opportunity to further the understanding, prevention or alleviation of a serious problem affecting the health and welfare of children."

Some ethicists, ourselves included, believe the federal regulations for *Research Involving Children* are too lenient insofar as nonbeneficial research is concerned. The main reason for this disagreement lies in the nature of proxy consent. A parent or guardian has the right of proxy consent only in order to benefit his or her child or ward. Although an adult may freely subject himself or herself to risk research in which there is no personal benefit, it seems that a parent or guardian does not have the same right over a child. Whatever the value of this opinion, it seems that the treatment given Baby Fae was unethical even if evaluated in light of the more liberal ethical norms contained in the federal regulations.

Discussion

In order to offer an ethical evaluation, let us ask the following questions:
1. Should the physicians who performed the transplant

on Baby Fae follow the federal guidelines for research on children? Legally speaking, they did not have to follow these guidelines because the research was funded by withholding a portion of the fees collected from private patients. (This method of funding research is an ethical issue in itself because cost shifting is involved.) Morally speaking, though, it seems that the researchers at Loma Linda University do have an obligation to follow the federal regulations because they offer minimal ethical standards for our pluralistic society. To put it another way, if researchers do not follow the federal norms, which ethical norms will they follow?

2. Did this research benefit Baby Fae directly or did it offer the kind of knowledge that would benefit other children? Despite some early enthusiastic statements from some of the physicians doing the transplant, there seems to be no doubt that the transplant was not of direct benefit to Baby Fae. Some might say, "Baby Fae benefitted because she would have died anyway and the transplant prolonged her life." But research may never be justified simply because the subject "will die anyway." Moreover, what benefit is it to prolong the life of an infant for three weeks and treat the infant as a thing rather than a person during that time? Others might say, "Maybe by some miracle she could have lived." But scientific research on human beings is not based on miracles, it is based on certified knowledge and previous research on animals. To say that the research did not benefit Baby Fae directly does not imply it was per se unethical, but it does mean that such research should be subject to stringent standards.

3. If the research did not benefit Baby Fae, did it involve more than minimal risk of harm? If so, was it a minor or a major increase? Clearly the surgery involved a major risk of harm. Not only was there the risk of immediate death, but there was the certainty of physical pain and suffering from the surgery and of deterioration of vital organs from the drugs used to suppress Baby Fae's immunological defenses. In addition to the risk of physical harm, the risk of emotional harm must be considered as well. Baby Fae spent her last days as a research object, not in the arms of a loving mother. In sum, it seems that the IRB at Loma Linda University did not have the right to approve the research on Baby Fae.

Conclusion

Because there was no hope of benefitting Baby Fae and because the risk of harm involved in the transplant procedure was a major increase over minimal harm, it seems that the baboon heart research proposal should have been submitted to a national panel of experts selected by the Secretary of Health and Human Services. Research involving transplants from animals is not in itself unethical, but it should be carried on only after the protocol, its scientific justification, and an analysis of risk and benefit have been evaluated and approved by a group of competent peers.

1. *Research Involving Children* (Washington, DC: National Commission for Protection of Human Subjects of Biomedical and Behavioral Research, OS77-0004, 1977); *Federal Register* vol. 48, n. 46 (Washington, DC: U.S. Government Printing Office, March 8, 1983); "Additional Protection for Children Involved as Subjects of Research," *Federal Register*, vol. 48, n. 46 (Washington, DC: U.S. Government Printing Office, March 8, 1983).

Advance Directives 48

In Missouri and other states there is legislation for "living wills," so-called natural death acts, or legislation and amendments of so-called durable power of attorney. The intention of this legislation is to ensure that patients who may eventually be incapable of giving directions about their health care will have a voice in the kind of treatment they refuse or accept. At first blush the legislation protects a patient's right of self-determination and provides security for the physician. Many people welcome this kind of legislation, and it may have its place; however, assurances that this legislation will protect the values of patient care may be too ambitious.

Assumptions

Underlying assumptions exist that give rise to the legislative attempts to pass natural death acts. The first assumption is that dying is a problem. It is a technical problem because of the highly technological care available. Patients perceive it as a problem because of what they read, see, and hear about the medical community. Physicians experience dying as a problem because of liability, a personal sense of failure, poor coping mechanisms, or institutional problems. Subsequently, the patient is kept "alive," and dying becomes a problem and answers to "the problem" are sought through the law. When should a person have a "right to die?" What social concerns require state intervention against people dying? Who makes these decisions?

The second assumption of living will legislation is that consensual cooperative dialogue between the patient, the physician, and the patient's family is difficult or impossible. As a result, consensual decisions made by the patient and the physician are questioned, and proxy decisions for incompetent patients are distrusted. Most disheartening, perhaps, is the assumption by some that physicians cannot be trusted, that they are unscrupulous and will not respond to patients' wishes and that something else is needed—preferably with enforceable punitive measures—to ensure their compliance with patients' wishes. Advance directives are an attempt by some patients to state their wishes clearly and by some physicians to be free of the unnecessary liability that can accompany medical decision making.

A third set of assumptions are really misconceptions about medicine, advance directives, and the law. The assumption is that statutory laws, such as the natural death act, will ensure appropriate decision making in medical care. They may preserve some of the patient's sense of self-determination, but such laws cannot ensure the fundamental values of the patient-provider relationship at the heart of medical care. Further, this legislation focuses on terminal illness, usually implying "imminent" death if treatment is withheld or withdrawn. Subjective preferences about treatment options for nonterminal situations for the noncompetent patient are not guaranteed. A stylized piece of legislation is not likely to promote communication which is the real value at stake. A law may reduce physician liability and promote patient autonomy in limited circumstances (and so should exist), but it will never ensure helpful communication (which is the heart of the problem). The underlying problems are difficult, and living wills may not resolve them. The living will may be a good indication of patient values as decisions are pondered, but it is not necessarily the key to decision making.

Discussion

Natural death acts and durable power of attorney acts seek to realize fundamental values in medicine. First, they attempt to secure the value of self-determination for the individual. Self-determination is an intelligent, comprehending, reflective process. Signing a living will because one fears what physicians and one's family will do does not necessarily realize that value. Openness to the wide variety of experiences and feelings that may affect one's choices, including the experience of illness, pain, and suffering, must also be respected if self-determination is to be realized.

Second, the value of the principle of allowing to die is

important. This requires reflection on the purpose of life and a willingness not to prolong dying or mere physical life. Respect for personal decisions about the burdensomeness of treatment is also at stake. More careful attention to the reality of death in life and the acceptance of death is as important as a living will.

The third value is that of open communication within the medical relationship. Good decisions about the withholding or the withdrawing of treatment are based on this dialogue between physicians and patients or their proxies. Often this communication is messy. Good interpersonal skills, in addition to well-drafted legislation, are needed.

A last issue that must be respected is the principle of proxy consent. One hopes that a proxy decision maker has the same information and the objectivity to make a decision for someone as the person would have made that decision. In this sense, the durable power of attorney act may have much more to offer than a natural death act.

It may be that natural death acts and other pieces of legislation are necessary; however, it still is imperative that the public and the medical community deal with the values that this legislation seeks to promote. First, the public needs more education. Wider appreciation for the latitude needed in medical decision making is necessary. In addition, the fact that illness affects different people in different ways must be stressed. This must be coupled with medical education for providers about death and dying, the value components of individual patients' decisions, and the tools necessary to listen well and respond appropriately to a patient or his or her proxy at a critical time.

Institutions also have an important role in educating the public. Both long-term and acute care facilities must seek ways to educate patients, to communicate patients' wishes, and to deal with family members who must make painful decisions. Only the cooperation of patient, family, provider, and institution will realize the patient values at stake in advance directives. A law may better provide for knowledgeable proxies to make a decision for an incompetent patient in accord with the patient's preferences. Also, a law may provide legal comfort for some providers. If so, fine. The legal sanctuary for physician and proxy, however, should never displace the central focus of the person and his or her values in medical decision making. For all its benefits, the living will may be too small to shoulder the many important values at stake in decisions to withhold or withdraw any kind of treatment.

"Few topics in medicine are more complicated, more controversial and more emotionally charged than treatment of the hopelessly ill."[1] So opine a group of physicians who nonetheless intrepidly attempt to offer other physicians guidelines for hopelessly ill adults in order "to come to some consensus about our responsibilities."[2] Because this document seems intended to serve as more than a guideline, its presuppositions and method deserve close scrutiny.

Principles

The panel presenting these guidelines for physicians is composed only of physicians. Have ethicists, theologians, or other health care professionals nothing to contribute? Sociological studies demonstrate that physicians have little training in ethics and hence take a pragmatic view whereby they value most an immediate practical solution. Hence unless they have formal education in the field, experience indicates that they need the help of ethicists in order to grasp the total problem and to solve it according to principle.

Rather than depend on ethical principles to substantiate their guidelines, physicians rely on the law or their own authority. Both the patient's right to make decisions about medical treatment and the physician's responsibility to refuse participation in suicide are substantiated in the article by the civil law. Law should be based on ethical principles. Thus there are more fundamental reasons than law for the aforementioned standards of patient consent and nonparticipation in suicide. Patients have a right to make decisions about their medical care because they must exercise freedom to fulfill their purpose in life. Physicians should not cooperate in suicide because human beings do not have absolute domination over their existence. Moreover, suicide destroys the bond of family and brings despair to society.

When the physicians reach the heart of the matter, stating the guidelines for withholding care, they do not even use the law as a basis of their statements. Rather, we are asked to accept the conclusions based on their personal authority. Hence although they use such words as "ethically permissible" and "morally justifiable," they do not offer any reasons for their statements. Medical ethics is a philosophical discipline, and in philosophy authority is the weakest of arguments. Thus, the physician's statements need more reasoned argumentation in their support.

Four levels of care are presented in the article: (1) emergency resuscitation; (2) intensive care and advanced life support; (3) general medical care, including antibiotics, drugs, surgery, cancer chemotherapy, artificial hydration, and nutrition; and (4) general nursing care and efforts to make the patient comfortable, including relief of pain, hydration, and nutrition as dictated by the patient's thirst and hunger. The spiritual and psychological needs, especially vital for dying patients, are not mentioned even as part of comfort care.

Two types of patients are discussed: those who are competent and those who are incompetent. Guidelines for the level of care for the competent patient focus on patient consent, relief from pain, emergency resuscitation, and hospice care. Incompetent patients are divided into patients with brain death, patients in a persistent vegetative state, severely and irreversibly demented patients, and elderly patients with permanent mild impairment of competence. Including the patient with brain death among incompetent patients only confuses the issue. Patients with brain death are not only "considered medically and legally dead." They *are* dead. If they are not dead in fact, then they must not be declared medically or legally dead.

Concerning patients in a persistent vegetative state, we are told that "it is morally justifiable to withhold antibiotics and artificial nutrition and hydration as well as other forms of life-sustaining treatment, allowing the patient to die."[3] Hence only the fourth level of care is necessary for these patients. As we have stated in a previous essay (see pages 65-68), we agree with this statement but ethical justification should be offered. The ethical justification for withholding life-prolonging care from a person in an irreversible persistent vegetative state is because the person can no longer strive effectively for the purpose of life. All medical care that aims at prolonging life is directed to helping people achieve the purpose of life. Although physicians and other health care professionals work at the level of psychiatric and physiological function, their work is ordered to the higher functions of the human person, which enables the person to strive for the purpose of life. All need not agree on the specific purpose of life; we define it in different ways. But all agree that when the higher functions can no longer operate, the person can no longer strive for the purpose of life; thus there is no need to prolong life.

The statement distinguishes between two types of demented patients: those severely and irreversibly demented and elderly patients with permanent mild impairment of competence. For the former group, only that care need be given to make them comfortable. "If such a patient rejects food and water by mouth, it is ethically permissible to withhold nutrition and hydration artificially administered by vein or gastric tube. It is ethically appropriate not to treat intercurrent illness except with measures required for comfort."[4] In regard to the second group, those who are "pleasantly senile," care should also be limited. In fact, if emergency resuscitation and intensive care are required, the physician should provide these measures sparingly. . .guided by the patient, or the patient's family, and by an assessment of the patient's prospects for improvement.[5]

Discussion

In a sense, the physicians seem to change the rules of the game when they discuss demented patients. Before this they discuss patients who are hopelessly ill *and* terminally ill and who have no potential to strive for the purpose of life. These demented patients are not terminally ill, however, nor are we sure that any individual is unable to strive for the purpose of life. Ethical reasoning also justifies allowing a person to die if prolonging life involves a grave burden in striving for the purpose of life. But this must be an individual judgment. It cannot be made of a class of people. In other words, we must be very sure that when discussing limitation of medical care we do not neglect the weak and suffering simply because they need our help. May we allow people to die simply because "they are a burden" or are supported by public funds? In a very real sense, each one of us has been or will be a "burden," and this should not imply that we are left to die. Stating that a person can freely choose to refuse aggressive treatment that would prolong life if the person is terminally ill is one thing; maintaining that one can make that same decision for a *class of people* when there is still a hope of a weak potential to strive for the purpose of life is completely different.

Conclusion

The meeting from which the document emanates was funded by the Society for the Right to Die. Although worthy of evaluation, the document should not stand as the last word on the matter.

1. Sidney H. Wagner, et al., "The Physicians' Responsibility Toward Hopelessly Ill Patients," *New England Journal of Medicine* 310 (1984): 955-959.
2. Wagner, p. 955.
3. Wagner, p. 955.
4. Wagner, p. 958.
5. Wagner, p. 958.

Mr. Bartling Is Dying: 50
Asking the Right Questions

William Bartling, aged seventy, was strapped to his bed at Glendale Adventist Medical Center in Los Angeles, CA, to prevent him from shutting off a ventilator and removing tubes from his throat, arms, or nose. The last six years of his life had been marked by declining health. On April 8, 1984, he was placed on a ventilator to ease his breathing after a diseased lung collapsed during a biopsy. Numerous attempts to wean him from the ventilator failed. Generally, the physicians agreed that he would not survive without the machines and that if the machines were stopped he would live only a few minutes. Mr. Bartling suffered from chronic emphysema, arteriosclerosis, heart disease, the ballooning of an artery section in his abdomen, and inoperable lung cancer.

Mr. Bartling's wife, Ruth, indicated that her husband no longer desired to be attached to the various devices. He has made a similar statement and said he understood he would die if his wish is honored. Mr. William Ginsburg, the hospital attorney, then asked if he would like to live, to which Mr. Bartling replied yes. Mr. Ginsburg contends that Mr. Bartling was therefore confused and questioned whether he is competent to make any medical decision. He declared, "He's alive and we are not going to let him die." The hospital was willing to transfer him, but no other institution would accept him. Richard Johnson, MD, his physician, stated that he was unwilling to withdraw any of the life-prolonging therapies.

The case went to court. Judge Lawrence Waddington of State Superior Court refused to order the withdrawal of treatment because although Mr. Bartling was terminally ill, his death was not imminent. The case was being appealed but in the meantime, Mr. Bartling died. Costs for care were estimated to be a half a million dollars, not including legal costs. The price of human pain and anxiety for all involved, especially Mr. Bartling and his family, cannot be quantified.

Principles and Discussion

The first ethical issue surrounds the question of whether, given Mr. Bartling's diagnosis and prognosis, it was permissible to allow him to die. Primacy in the legal opinion was given to the withdrawal of therapies rather than to the possibility of Mr. Bartling pursuing the purpose of life. If the treatments given promoted mere physiological life with no realistic ability to pursue the ends of life in even a minimal fashion, or if the therapies merely sustained certain bodily functions until thorough breakdown occurred, then it is Mr. Bartling's dying and not his living that was being prolonged. Asking and answering questions in a logically ordered fashion is crucial to resolving this problem. The question of allowing to die precedes the question of the withdrawal of a therapy.

Second, informed consent and competency are not to be judged solely by the patient's wish to live or by the category of disease. It is very possible that Mr. Bartling would like to have continued living but also realized the fruitlessness of the medical treatment. His statement that he wanted the machines turned off, realizing that he would die, while still affirming a basic drive to live, was not necessarily an indication of incompetency. Criteria used for competency decisions can and often do involve ambiguity. The basic question remains: Did Mr. Bartling understand his disease and the consequences of the various alternatives to treatment, including refusing further treatment?

Third, Judge Waddington's concern about the imminence of death is simply too narrow from the ethical perspective. Allowing a person to die, and subsequently the withdrawal and withholding of treatment, can be done either because of the imminence of death, because of the burden of treatment to the patient, or because the therapy is useless in promoting the basic goods of health and the purpose of life. At a time when medicine has the technology to stave off death for prolonged periods, it is necessary to examine carefully whether the lack of imminence of death is due to the presence and possibility of life or to the prolongation of dying. Because burdens vary between different patients, it is important to account for these carefully. Prolonged intensive care and multiple tubes and machines may well have been a serious burden for Mr. Bartling, even if the physician or the hospital's lawyer does not think so. Imminence is not the only ethical criteria.

Fourth, the sacredness of life referred to by the attorney was congruent with the traditional values, goals, and purposes of medicine. Sacredness of life is not consistent with vitalism, however. Protecting the dignity and sacredness of life is not promoted when the final process of living, one's dying, is not treated with respect. Nuances, difficult as they are, must be considered in the sacredness of life ethic.

Fifth, a hospital has the right and the obligation to uphold certain values consistent with its religious traditions, but even these values are developed within a patient-centered perspective. The trepidation expressed by the hospital in this area of dying and when confronted by difficult legal issues is understandable. When legal issues predominate, however, it is too easy to forget that ethical issues are the foundation of law. Too often it is the patient who loses. Mr. Bartling's case and others are too complex to find their resolution in legal precedent alone. Hospitals have an important commitment to patients and their health care that cannot be undermined by legal intricacies. Risks are always a part of medical treatment. Hospital administrators must clarify the main objective of their institutions and ensure that patient care is not compromised by legal entanglements.

Last, money is an issue. It would be unethical if only those with money received medical care. There is not an unending money supply for health care, however; allocating financial resources while making sound ethical decisions is a difficult part of health care decisions. When there are many competing claims for health care dollars, it is important to ensure that money is not wasted in unnecessary or useless care. These are difficult but necessary decisions.

Conclusion

A person's health care at the time of death is a concern of medicine, health care institutions, and health care law. Mr.

Bartling's personal values and desires, however, cannot be forgotten or made secondary to the related questions of contemporary technology or the law. The ethical, medical, and legal questions that technology raises can be answered only when we ask the right questions and reason carefully from those responses.

A Broadway play entitled *Whose Life Is It Anyway?*, by Brian Clark, has portrayed dramatically the problem of what type of care to give people who may be kept alive in a conscious state but whose level of human activity is drastically impaired.[1] This problem is solved rather easily when the person in question is elderly, in an irreversible coma, and near death from natural causes. Then there is little question that life-supporting means may be removed and "nature allowed to take its course." But when the person concerned is conscious and states that he or she does not wish to live an impaired life with mechanical support systems, what judgment should be made? *Whose Life Is It Anyway?* offers a means to consider this problem.

The Characters

Ken Harrison is a young sculptor who has had a very serious automobile accident. Six months after the accident, he is still in the hospital, and "as a result of treatment, all the broken bones and ruptured tissues have healed and all that remains is the ruptured spinal column and the mental trauma." Because he will be paralyzed for the rest of his life, unable to care for himself in any way, Ken decides that he does not wish to go on living. When informed by a social worker of the things he will be able to do "with training and a little patience," such as operate a typewriter and reading machines, he replies that this "would not be good enough." When discussing the situation with his lawyer, Ken states that although he realizes that other people may live with dire handicaps, for him, life would be too burdensome if he were to continue in this way. Ken, then, wishes to be discharged from the hospital, and have the catheter removed so that "the toxic substances will build up in the bloodstream and poison him."

Dr. Emerson, the attending physician, believes that Ken is merely depressed and that if given more time will choose to live. He states, "It is impossible to injure the body to the extent that Mr. Harrison has and not affect the mind." From his experience, he thinks that Ken will change his mind later on. In order to prevent Ken's discharge and ensuing death, Dr. Emerson seeks to have Ken committed to the hospital as mentally unstable, but Ken's lawyers apply for a writ of *habeas corpus*, which would free Ken to leave the hospital and discontinue the lifesaving care. The climax of the play is the hearing on the writ of *habeas corpus*, Justice Millhouse presiding.

The Plot

Does Ken have the moral right to choose death in this situation? Is he committing suicide? For solving this problem, ethicists use the principle of ordinary and extraordinary means. If the catheter is judged to be an extraordinary means, then it may be removed and thus Ken would be allowed to die. From an ethical point of view, a surgical procedure, medical device, or medicine cannot be determined as ordinary or extraordinary until we know the patient's condition and whether prolonging life will help the person attain the goal of life. Ordinary means, then, are those that do not involve a grave burden for oneself or another, judged according to the circumstances of persons, places, times, and cultures; extraordinary means do involve a grave burden. Another means of determining whether means are ordinary or extraordinary is to ask, "Will prolonging life through this means present an intolerable burden to the patient," or "Will prolonging life make it too difficult to achieve the goal of life?"

The reason why we can make the distinction between ordinary and extraordinary means from an ethical point of view is because human life is not the greatest good, nor the greatest value. Life, health, and all temporary activities are subordinated to spiritual ends. True, human life is a very important gift that we should protect and foster. We have a duty toward God, as well as toward other people, to protect our life and health, but in some cases, protecting or prolonging human life may not contribute to achieving that more important good, the purpose of human life. People may differ in defining the purpose of human life. Some may describe it as sapient life, others as the potential to relate to others, and others as spiritual growth and development. All seem to agree, though, that when the purpose can no longer be achieved, the duty to prolong life is no longer present. That is why a respirator may be judged as an extraordinary means for a person in an irreversible coma, and that is why a person with a terminal illness may determine that trying to cure the illness is worse than dying now. In Ken's case, he seems to be saying that the pain and suffering associated with his disabilities make it too burdensome for him to prolong life. In effect, he is saying, "Insofar as achieving the goal of life is concerned, it would be less burdensome to let me die now than to prolong the pain and suffering through such medical means as a catheter."

The Last Act

To find out what Justice Millhouse, Dr. Emerson, and Ken finally decide, see or read the play. All in all, we do not think that Ken is asking to commit suicide; rather, he is asking to be allowed to die. But we agree with Dr. Emerson that Ken should have some time to think over the situation and experience the type of life he would be able to lead as an invalid before the catheter is removed. Life is sweet, and not many people really wish to die. In this regard, a physician stated recently:

> Talk about a "dignified death" usually comes from onlookers, not from the patient. Most patients want to live. . . Dignity lies in their fight for life and in their struggle to maintain contact with humanity. Kindness, personal attention, and good nursing help to preserve a patient's dignity.[2]

1. B. Clark, *Whose Life Is It Anyway?*, (Chicago: The Dramatic Publishing Company, 1974).
2. Franklin H. Epstein, "Responsibility of the Physician in the Preservation of Life," *Archives of Internal Medicine* (1979): 919.

Determination of Death: 52
An Ethical Analysis of Legislation

Since 1970, over thirty states have passed laws allowing the determination of death through lack of brain function. The laws differ among states, but, in general, they allow a physician to declare that human death has occurred when the clinical signs of irreversible and complete cessation of total brain functions are present and respiration and circulation are maintained artificially. The main reasons for this legislation are to dispose for successful organ transplants and to protect physicians from irresponsible malpractice litigation.

Principles

In order to analyze the ethical validity of these laws, several facts must be kept in mind:

1. The term *definition of death* legislation is a misnomer. What we are concerned with is the legal right for a physician to make a declaration of death from signs associated with complete and irreversible cessation of brain functions.

2. There are two distinct questions involved:

a. Is there a set of signs, medically substantiated, that can be used to declare that human death has occurred when the traditional signs (irreversible cessation of spontaneous respiration and circulation) cannot be discerned because a respirator is used? This question, to be answered primarily by physicians but with the help of philosophers, has been answered in the affirmative.

b. Should physicians be given the legal right to use the signs in question, usually referred to as the brain death syndrome, when declaring the fact of human death? This is a question to be answered by legislators after having consulted physicians, others in the profession of health care, and those who might be affected by such legislation.

3. Declaring human death from the signs associated

with brain death syndrome presupposes that a respirator is in use and that the traditional clinical signs of human death (i.e., irreversible cessation of spontaneous functions of heart and lungs) are not observable. The declaration of human death from the signs of brain death implies, however, that the more traditional signs of human death would soon appear if the respirator were removed.

4. From a medical point of view, the signs used to determine that human death has occurred should have the following qualities:

a. *clear*— that is, not ambiguous, not dependent on mere opinion, and in accord with the known physiology of the living human person.

b. *certain*— that is, taken together, the signs must give conclusive proof of human death; the dying person must be given the benefit of any doubt.

c. *irreversible*— that is, medical experience and documentation must testify conclusively that people (the bodily remains of people) in this condition do not regain the signs of human life.

5. Some physicians and philosophers maintain that human death occurs if there are certain signs that only partial brain death (dysfunction of the cerebral cortex only) has occurred[1] Whether this is a sufficient sign of human death is not at question here. The legislation enacted in the various states has not sought to approve the declaration of death using signs of partial brain death. Rather, this legislation seeks to recognize signs of total brain death; that is, signs that indicate that a complete and irreversible cessation of all brain functions has occurred. With this in mind, the set of signs used by physicians, and the language of the legislation, must be signs and language that indicate that human death already has occurred, not that it will occur shortly if the same signs perdure. Although some dispute this point, it seems that the safer methodology should be followed in this most serious of human decisions.[2]

Discussion

In general, legislation should not be enacted unless it promotes or enforces ethical obligations or rights that would not otherwise be observed sufficiently. In order to discuss the need for legal recognition of the brain death syndrome, then, we must delineate the major ethical obligations and rights involved in this issue. They seem to be as follows:

1. One should not declare that a person has died until clear, certain, and irreversible signs show that the lifegiving principle (often called the soul) no longer informs (enlivens and organizes) the remains of the human being in question.

2. One should treat the remains of a human being with respect.

3. One should be willing to enhance life for other people provided the action does not violate other serious ethical obligations. Usually, then, one should be willing to allow one's vital organs to be transplanted to another person after death.

4. One should be able to practice medicine and offer health care without fear of irresponsible malpractice accusations and litigation.

In theory, the above ethical rights could be respected, and the above obligations could be fulfilled, without a state law. But, in practice, it seems a state law is necessary to guarantee fulfillment of these major rights and obligations. Whatever the extrinsic political motives for this legislation, the ethical issues outlined above should be the focal point in passing or rejecting brain death legislation.

1. Robert Rizzo and Paul Yonder, "Definition and Criteria of Clinical Death," *Linacre Quarterly*, 40(1973): 223-233; DeMere McCarthy, "Hearing Before the Missouri Senate Select Committee on the Definition of Death," Sept. 10, 1976.
2. Paul Byrne, Sean O'Reilly, and Paul Quay, "Brain Death: An Opposing Viewpoint," *Journal of the American Medical Association* 242(1979): 1985-1990.

Tube Feeding— 53
Routine Nursing Care?

In 1984, two physicians in California were charged with felony murder because they withdrew life-support systems from a brain-damaged patient. Because there was no hope of the patient's recovery, with permission of the family, the physicians removed the respirator. When the patient continued breathing without assistance, tubes feeding him nourishment and water were also removed. Six days later, the patient died. In California a preliminary hearing is held before a murder trial to determine whether sufficient evidence exists to proceed with the trial. At the preliminary hearing the judge determined that the evidence was insufficient and dismissed the criminal case.

At present, removing a respirator from a comatose patient who will not recover has been accepted as standard and ethical practice in medicine. But removing artificial methods of providing food and water when the patient is in the same condition is not so readily accepted. In 1983 a physician, recounting in the *New England Journal of Medicine* his problems of conscience in caring for elderly people stated, "In our nursing home, for example, there is a middle-aged woman who has been comatose for five years as a result of an accident. Although there is no meaningful chance that she will ever improve, she is certainly not "brain dead" and is supported *only* by *routine nursing care* that consists of tube feedings, regular turnings, urinary catheters, and good hygiene; she is on no respirator or other machine" [emphasis added].[1] For some medical professionals, then, tube feeding patients who are in an irreversible coma is considered standard and proper treatment. But is this an ethical conclusion? Has the practice of using tube feeding, regular antibiotics to avoid infection, and urinary catheters resulted from an ethical analysis of the situation or from a false supposition that physicians must "do everything possible?"

Principles

Medicine aims at preventing sickness, restoring health, and prolonging life. About this there can be no mistake. But ethical health care professionals realize that they must prolong life in a manner consistent with the patient's value system and the ethical standards of medicine. In the value system upon which medical care is based, prolonging the life of a person who is irreversibly comatose is not considered a value for the patient or the physician.[2] Mere physiological existence is not a value if no potential for mental-creative function exists. True, it is often difficult to determine if a coma is irreversible. When there is a reasonable doubt about the patient's condition, and some hope that he or she might recover, prolonging life through life-support systems is indicated. But if a reasonable doubt does not exist, then the ethical decision is to let the patient die. When this decision has been made, the goal is to keep the patient as comfortable as possible. To this end, analgesics may be given, even if they indirectly shorten life.[3]

Discussion

When the decision has been made to allow the patient to die, does providing nourishment and water through tubes constitute a life-support system or is it a means of keeping the patient comfortable? Hydration of some type seems necessary to keep a person comfortable. If tube feeding is the only way to accomplish this, then it seems to be in order. But is nourishment required? In many cases the patient is actually dying of a malfunction of the digestive system, and this malfunction is obviated by a life-support system such as tube feeding. It seems then that tube feeding could be withdrawn from a patient when a decision has been made to let him or her die, because this is a life-support system rather than a comfort device. If the objection is raised that the patient may suffer hunger or "starve to death," two responses are in order: (1) the pain may be alleviated through analgesics; and (2) the patient is not starving to death but is dying of a malfunction of the digestive system and it is time to let nature take its course.

Perhaps the effect of tube feeding will be understood more clearly if we compare it to the use of the respirator. When a decision has been made to allow a patient to die and the respirator is removed, the patient will die of lack of oxygen (lack of cardiopulmonary function). Ethically, the decision to remove the respirator is justified because there is no longer any responsibility to prolong life. In like manner, nourishment by artificial means may be removed. The patient will die because he cannot assimilate food by natural function, just as the person on the respirator cannot assimilate oxygen by natural function. What has been said about the respirator and tube feeding is true of other life-support efforts once a decision has been made to allow the patient to die.

If tube feeding can be withheld from an elderly person after a decision has been made that life need not be prolonged, why not allow the withholding of food from a newborn with Down's syndrome and claim that it would die of natural causes? To withhold food from a Down's syndrome child would be unethical because it is the natural process for infants to receive food from others. A Down's syndrome child is not dying of a pathological digestive system. Moreover, making a decision that a child should be allowed to die merely because he or she has Down's syndrome is unethical because the child has the potential for mental-creative function.

Would not this interpretation of tube feeding for comatose patients cause undue concern if publicized by health care professionals? Yes, probably it would. For this reason, it is the responsibility of ethicists to make known that once the decision has been made to allow a patient to die, only comfort therapy is in order. Twenty-five years ago many people did not accept withdrawal of a respirator as "standard practice." Now it is accepted as ethical medical practice when the decision has been made to allow the patient to die. Through discussion in the public forum, the same acceptance would develop in regard to tube feeding and other procedures.

Conclusion

In light of the limited resources and some trends in health care, we must make sure that people are not allowed to die merely because they are elderly. On the other hand, we must also provide that the lives of elderly people are not extended unduly because the people involved, families and health care professionals, are hesitant to make accurate ethical decisions.

1. David Hilfiker, "Allowing the Debilitated to Die," *New England Journal of Medicine* 308(1983): 716-719.
2. For more on the ethics of allowing a person to die, see Kevin O'Rourke, "Allowing a Person to Die," in *Critical Care, State of the Art*, 3(1983): 1-27.
3. Vincent Collins, "Managing Pain and Prolonging Life," *New Technologies of Birth and Death* (St. Louis: Pope John XXIII Medical-Moral Research and Education Center, 1980): 144-149.

The Claire Conroy Case: 54
Withholding Tube Feeding

Claire Conroy, an eighty-four-year-old patient in a long-term care facility, suffered from severe organic brain syndrome, necrotic decubitus ulcers, urinary tract infection, arteriosclerotic heart disease, hypertension, and diabetes mellitus. She was unable to speak or move, although from her fetal position she sometimes followed people with her eyes. Nurses were not able to feed her by hand, so a nasogastric tube was inserted and several times a day a nutrient formula, vitamins, and medicine were poured through the tube. Her only surviving relative, her nephew and legal guardian, requested the Superior Court of Essex County, NJ, to allow the nasogastric tube to be removed and thus allow Claire Conroy to die. The Superior Court granted the request, but the Appellate Division of New Jersey reversed the lower court's decision. The Supreme Court of New Jersey decided to review the decision of the appellate court even though Claire Conroy had died with the tube in place in the meantime because of the relevance for other people in long-term care facilities and hospitals in the same condition. On Jan. 17, 1985, the decision of the Supreme Court of New Jersey became public, and because this decision (like the Karen Ann Quinlan decision from the same court) will have ethical and legal ramifications for the whole country, we shall consider the pertinent statements and assumptions of the decision in this essay. All quotes, unless noted otherwise, are from the New Jersey Supreme Court decision.[1]

Principles

The court decided that "life-sustaining treatment may be withheld from incompetent patients when it can be determined that the patient would have refused the treatment under the circumstances involved." The proof that a person would have refused life-prolonging treatment in such circumstances "may have been expressed orally, or in writing, or it might be deduced from a person's religious belief or prior decisions about medical care."

The same decision may be made for incompetent patients whose desires about treatment cannot be determined "if it is manifest that such action would further the patient's best interest." In these latter cases, how does the surrogate determine "the best interests of the patient"? The court answers the question by stating that a limited objective or a pure objective test should be used, depending on knowledge of the patient's desires. "Under the *limited objective test* . . . there is some trustworthy evidence (but not a clear expression) that the patient would have refused the treatment and the decisionmaker is satisfied that the burdens of the patient's continued life with the treatment outweighs the benefits of life for him." In the *pure objective test* there is no evidence of the patient's desire, but the life support treatment may be removed, if "the net burdens of the patient's life with the treatment should clearly and markedly outweigh the benefits that the patient derives from life."

How does the court define an incompetent patient? "A patient is incompetent if medical evidence establishes that the patient is an elderly incompetent nursing home resident with severe and permanent mental and physical impairments and a life expectancy of approximately one year or less." A few comments about this description are in order. Why must the patient be elderly? Ethically speaking, the same standards should be used for all patients. The statement in regard to the time the patient will live seems superfluous. Even if life expectancy with tube feeding would be more than one year, the ethical standards for removing the tube feeding could still be present.

Discussion

The court explained its standards by stating the following:

We expressly decline to authorize

decision based on assessments of personal worth, or social utility of another's life of the value of that life to others. We do not believe that it should be appropriate for a court. . . to determine that someone else's life is not worth living simply because the patient's 'quality of life' or value to society seems negligible. The mere fact that a patient's functioning is limited or his prognosis dim does not mean that he is not enjoying the remains of his life or that it is in his best interest to die.

The court explains the burden-benefit ratio by declaring, "By this we mean that the patient is suffering, and will continue to suffer, unavoidable pain and that the net burdens of prolonged life markedly outweigh any physical pleasure, emotional enjoyment or intellectual satisfaction that the patient may be able to derive from life."

Summarizing these statements, we can delineate three conditions that must be present in order to withhold or withdraw tube feeding from an incompetent patient: (1) a terminal pathological condition is prevented by tube feeding; (2) the patient's overall condition is such that he or she cannot strive for the social or spiritual (creative) values of life even with the tube feeding; and (3) the condition is judged medically irreversible. By this decision, tube feeding may be considered the same as a respirator or any other mechanical device that prevents a physical pathological condition from causing death (see also pages 212-215).

Care should be taken to ensure that the patient does not suffer pain because tube feeding is not used. Thus hydration or analgesics might be used to keep a patient comfortable as death approaches. The court's decision does not countenance withholding food and water from patients who are able to eat, even if such nourishment must be prepared and given to them by others.

The court allows tube feeding and other treatment to be continued for persons in Claire Conroy's condition, no matter how great the burden, "if the patient expressed the desire to be kept alive in spite of any pain that he might experience." This seems to be an unreasonable statement because it approves the effort to maintain life after the point at which a person can no longer strive for values and purpose of life. Mere physical existence is not a human value, and a person's wishes should not be allowed to circumvent the reasonable practice of medicine. Medical care is unethical if it is useless care.[2]

Conclusion

With a few reservations then, the basis for the Claire Conroy decision seems to be ethically sound. One would hope that it disposes physicians and families to realize that the goal in care for the dying is to help the patient die well, not to extend mere physical existence.

---

1. In the Matter of Claire Conroy, New Jersey Supreme Court, 486 A.2d, 1209(Jan. 1985).
2. G. Annis, "From Quinlan to Conroy," *Hastings Center Report*, 15(April 1985): 24-26.

In May, 1977, a bill intended to increase the supply of corneal tissue available for transplants was debated in the Missouri State Senate. The bill (SB 577) allows "a coroner, or coroner's physician, to remove eye tissue of a decedent upon request of an eye bank. . .in any case in which a patient needs a transplant of corneal tissue," provided:

1. "That the decedent having suitable eye tissue for transplant is under his jurisdiction;

2. No contrary indication as to the disposition of the eye was given by the decedent or his declared next of kin; and

3. Removal of the eye will not interfere with the course of an investigation or autopsy."

The bill also states that "neither the coroner, the coroner's physician, nor the eye bank receiving the corneal tissue may be held liable in any civil or criminal action for failure to obtain consent of the next of kin before removing corneal tissue for transplant purposes."

Principles

Although the bill did not pass the Senate, it offers some ethical issues for consideration concerning the retrieval of organs from cadavers even if the people did not request retrieval of their organs when alive. Two issues were involved in this discussion: one is political; the other, ethical. The political issues might be stated in this way: What is the most effective way to obtain corneal tissue from the deceased—through a voluntary effort that persuades people to will their eyes or other organs for the use of others, or through a legislative effort that allows the tissue to be taken from a decedent provided no opposition has been expressed by the person when alive or by a next of kin after death? Until now, the voluntary effort was thought sufficient, and for this reason the Anatomical Gift Act has been recognized in all fifty states.[1] Insofar as the political question is concerned, definite evidence is needed before legislators contemplate retrieval of organs without the decedents' permission.

If the need for legislation is affirmed, then the ethical question must be considered. It might be phrased in this manner: Do the remains of a human person deserve any special respect that would preclude harvesting organs even if the decedent did not request such actions?

Although the remains of the human body may resemble the body of a living person, and although this resemblance may be prolonged through embalming, the remains are not a *human* body, but, rather, a mass of matter decomposing into constitutive, organic elements. If the corpse is not a *human* body, then why be concerned about the respect or reverence it receives? Respect and reverence are due the remains of a human being because of the sacredness of the human life that once informed the now decomposing mass. Respect for a dead body signifies respect for human life, respect for the person who now exists in another modality, respect for the author of life, and respect for the decedent's relatives.

Hence respect for the remains of the deceased person has meaning beyond its apparent signification. The practice of respecting the remains of a human being is a cross-cultural phenomenon, being found in the most ancient and primitive civilizations as well as today. Practices of this nature seem to fulfill the human need to demonstrate love as well as grief.

Discussion

In order to show due respect for the remains of a person, then, no organs should be removed from the corpse unless sufficient reason exists. To help a living person benefit from the remains of a deceased person is certainly a noble and sufficient reason to allow an organ or other tissue to be removed from the corpse.[2] From an ethical point of view, then, willing one's organs "to science" or for the benefit of some unknown person is considered to be a good action. But because the remains of a person in some way signify the person, if a person before death states, for religious or other reasons, that he opposes having his organs transplanted, this wish should be observed. In like manner, because the next of kin are thought to reflect accurately the wishes of the deceased, their desire should be followed too.

What should be done, however, if the person, while alive, expressed no preference on this matter? Does the state have the right to say that approval should be assumed? It seems reasonable to say that the person who died without making a statement denying permission for retrieval of organs could be presumed to agree with a procedure that benefits another human being. Presumptions of this nature by which we interpret the mind of another are made frequently (e.g., in the case of unconscious or comatose people). Thus it is ethical to presume what a person might wish to have done provided valid grounds for the presumption exists. Presuming that a deceased person would not object if organs or tissue from his or her remains would benefit another person is reasonable and just, even though the donation actually was not made.

The same presumption could be made ethically in regard to the next of kin, provided they are unavailable for consultation. Although the next of kin do not "own" the remains of the deceased, respect for the decedent requires that, if possible, they should be consulted and their wishes followed. But if they are not available, the presumption of permission is ethically sound. In the United States, few states have laws allowing this presumption, but it is the accepted norm in European countries.

---

1. The Anatomical Gift Act is "designed to facilitate the donation and use of human tissue and organs for transplantation and other medical purposes and provide a favorable legal environment for such activities." Alfred Sadler, et al., "The Uniform Anatomical Gift Act," *Journal of the American Medical Association* 206(1968): 2501-2506.
2. P. Ramsey, *The Patient As Person* (New Haven: Yale University Press, 1970): p. 198.

"On Selling Organs"   56

Given the shortage of human organs for transplants, should we advocate an open market on kidneys, or even hearts, or whatever organs may be transplantable in the immediate future? Should we allow people to sell their organs, even if it means death to the donor, under the assumption that we cannot stop a person from disposing of his or her assets? Some people believe "people have a right to sell their organs as portions of their bodies. . . because no one has a right to stop them from disposing of their assets as they will."[1] In order to consider this question from an ethical point of view, three questions must be considered:

1. Can we justify transplants from one living person to another?

2. Should one sell an organ for transplant?

3. Should there be laws against selling organs for transplant?

Principles

Can we justify transplants between living persons? Two types of transplants are possible: one involving an organ or tissue taken from a dead person and given to a living person; and the other involving an organ taken from a living person and given to another living person. When an organ is taken from a dead person and given to a living person, the transplant itself does not pose an ethical issue. If an ethical issue does arise, it stems from another source; for example, is the donor truly dead?

Ethical issues, however, are directly involved in transplants between living people. When the question of organ transplants between living persons was first discussed, many physicians and philosophers thought it was wrong. They had some good reasons for their position. Before this time, the only reason for removing an organ from the human body was disease or malfunction of the organ that seriously endangered total body function. As a surgeon might put it, one does not have the right to mutilate a healthy body. The ethical way of expressing this argument, based on the principle of totality, is to say that the integrity of the body should not be sacrificed unless there is a serious physiological danger to the whole body.

One of the pioneers in the field of bioethics, however, Rev. Gerald Kelly, SJ, long associated with Saint Louis University, added another idea to the debate concerning transplants. He pointed out that anatomical integrity of the body is not the same as functional integrity, and at times we might sacrifice anatomical integrity without sacrificing functional integrity. If an arm were transplanted there would be a loss of functional as well as anatomical integrity, a kidney being transplanted sacrifices anatomical integrity but maintains functional integrity because one kidney can serve the needs of the entire body. True, some future risk may be foreseen if the donor's other kidney should malfunction, but this type of potential risk is present even if the transplant does not occur. The risk of future difficulty might be a bit greater, but it is not of a different nature. In order to justify the risk and the loss of anatomical integrity that does occur, Fr. Kelly posited that the motivation for the donor should be charity, that is, the love of a fellow human being. Paul Ramsey, another pioneer in the field of bioethics, added that the common good of the community would be enhanced by the love the donor displayed. Organ donation is not an obligation in justice then; rather, it is choosing to be charitable. Moreover, a healthy human organ is much more than "an asset to be bought or sold." It is an integral part of the human personality and should not be sacrificed unless functional integrity is maintained and proper motivation is present.

Should one sell an organ for transplant? If the justification for donating an organ should be charity, then it seems contradictory to state that ethically one could sell his or her organ. The anatomical integrity of the human being is a great good and should be sacrificed only for the highest of motives. Moreover, moral chaos would ensue if organs were sold to the highest bidder. One might argue that a person in dire poverty may need the money that would come from an organ donation to support his or her family. If a person is indigent, other ways should be made available for his or her support.

Some might object that because people are paid for their blood, they should be paid for their organs as well. There is a difference between donating blood, which the body replaces, and donating an organ, which is not replaced. There is less risk in giving blood, and hence it could be justified with a less lofty monetary motive. It does seem, though, that the nation would be better served if people were not paid for blood donations. Rather than offer a motivation of money, the motivation of helping other people should be offered. A general education campaign could be instigated to encourage people to donate blood periodically. In sum, buying or selling human organs is unethical because it is contrary to the dignity of the human being and because need, rather than wealth, should determine who receives an organ.

Should there be a law against selling organs? If ethical rights and obligations are being observed in society, no law is needed. At present, no commercial traffic in human organs exists, and therefore a law does not seem necessary. If immunization problems are overcome in the future, transplants will increase, and there might be more tendency to sell organs. Even if this happens, though, would it be better to depend on the integrity and ethical value system of the medical profession to guarantee that the present system is maintained rather than depend upon laws? Through education and emphasis on the help that one person should offer another, it seems that enough organs would be donated and the proper ethical values maintained.[2] At the same time, as education on organ donations continues, some thought should be given to reversing the methods by which blood is obtained. Even selling blood seems contrary to the charity we should have for one another.

1. J. Lachs, "On Selling Organs," *Forum on Medicine* (Nov. 1979): 746-747.
2. Recently, the federal government prohibited the sale of human organs as part of a plan to increase the availability and reasonable allotment of human organs. The National Organ Transplant Act, PL 98-507; Cong. Record, Oct. 19, 1984.

Who Shall Live?   57

In 1983, a two-year-old child in Massachusetts was dying of a diseased liver. Her father, a hospital administrator, spoke at a convention of pediatricians, requesting that they keep his child in mind if they encountered a potential liver donor. The request received significant publicity, and the parents of another dying child in Colorado specified that after death their child's liver be donated to the child in Massachusetts. The transplantation seems to have been successful.

We rejoice with the parents of the child whose life was prolonged. But imagine that your child had been waiting for a liver transplant for a longer time than the child in Massachusetts. How would you feel if your child's opportunity to live had been sacrificed because other parents had been able to gain more publicity for the plight of their child?

Principles

In the immediate future a dramatic increase in the ability to transplant human organs and an even more dramatic increase in the demand for human organs will occur. Kidney transplants have become rather commonplace, but hearts, lungs, and livers are also being transplanted. Moreover, experiments are underway in animals to pave the way for transplantation of the small bowel and the grafting of adrenal gland tissues into the human brain for the treatment of Parkinson's disease. How will we as a society handle this demand? Will we allow or encourage a free market or a black market to develop for the sale of human organs? Recently a woman in Rock Island, suffering from heart disease, offered to sell one of her kidneys for $20,000. In Brazil, advertisements appear daily in newspapers offering corneas, kidneys, and blood for sale. Scientists, physicians, and ethicists have agreed that donation of organs should proceed from a charitable, not a monetary, motive. This conviction stems from a realization that the donation of an organ is, in a certain sense, a donation of life and therefore is above monetary value. Moreover, if organs were sold to the highest bidder, then the wealthy would have first choice, and this is contrary to the principles on which our society rests. Thomas Cooper, MD, president of the St. Louis Metropolitan Medical Society, believes that the Red Cross should be responsible for collecting and distributing vital organs, as it is for collecting and distributing blood. Although this is a valuable suggestion, vital questions still remain. What ethical norms will the Red Cross use in determining the recipients of vital organs, and who will make the decisions?

Discussion

As a step in providing some ethical norms for selecting organ recipients, the following thoughts are put forward:

1. All persons in dire need of organ donation should be enrolled in a regional organ donation center. Physicians or transplant teams would be requested to work through the center.

2. Because the purpose of the transplant is to prolong life for as long as possible, an attempt must be made to judge both the *need* of the transplant and the potential for *success*. Those more in danger of death would receive a higher priority (need), but among these, those with potential for better survival (success) would be chosen first. Patients would not be disqualified because of age alone; however, because age often presages development of complications after surgery, an older patient would be given a lower priority than a younger person in the same general physical condition. The etiology of the disease should also be considered, because a person who is in need of a liver transplant because of alcoholism or a person in need of a lung transplant because of smoking would not be as good a health risk as persons whose difficulties resulted from other causes.

3. The person's contribution to society must be taken into consideration as well; otherwise, there is danger that people with money, prestige, or higher education automatically would be considered more worthy candidates. In a democratic

society, where all in theory are equal, there might be a tendency to eliminate consideration of worth to society; however, there is some justice in trying to save the father of a family instead of an unmarried person, if all other criteria are equal. Hence one's position in a family and one's actual and potential contribution to society should be considered.

4. If candidates seem to be equal in other criteria, then those who register first should be given higher priority. Hence this criterion would not be the most important but would be considered if the others do not offer a clear classification of candidates.

5. At present, permission of family, spouse, or legal guardian is required in order to harvest organs for transplant from a cadaver. (In the future, as transplantation becomes more successful and common, our laws on this matter may change.) Allowing the family, spouse, or legal guardian to specify the person who will receive the organs, however, does not seem fitting. Certain donations of organs among living members of a family should be allowed, but having the family or spouse of the dead person specify the recipient could defeat the ethical purpose of a selection system.

6. After attempting to classify people according to the above criteria, doubt may still exist on the best candidate. If so, then final selection from among those with highest priority should be made by lot. Although this does not provide that the ultimate choice will be made in accord with reasoned principles, it does provide that unfair and prejudicial standards will not predominate in the final selection.

7. Who will make these decisions that not even Solomon would have attempted? When in doubt, organize a committee. The talents needed to make fair decisions would require people with different skills and sensitivities, and so four or five people would be called on to work as volunteers under the sponsorship of the Red Cross.

Conclusion

As medical knowledge and technique make it possible to prolong the lives of more people, we are forced to make choices. Choices always involve value decisions. Unless we have agreed on norms and standards for our value decisions, we foster injustice, violence, and anarchy. Hence in the matter of determining norms for recipients of organ transplantation, we are discussing something of more than casual concern.

Medicine, Technology, and Health Care   58

At 4:09 am on Dec. 3, 1984, in the University of Utah Medical Center, Barney Clark, DDS, a sixty-one-year-old retired dentist suffering from cardiomyopathy, became the first recipient of an artificial heart called the Jarvik-7. The operation marked another breakthrough in medical science and technology, raising the hopes of many other heart patients who suffer from this and other heart diseases. Even though Barney Clark died about six weeks after the artificial heart was installed, a series of ethical questions was raised by this procedure. Among the most pertinent questions are those related to the development of technology as opposed to other values in health care, the assumptions about death in high-technology development, allowing people to die versus issues of suicide, and quality of life issues raised by the scarcity of medical resources and the cost of high technology.

Principles

There are different nuances in the use of the word *technology*. Technology can refer to an object—an artificial heart, which was placed in Dr. Clark's chest through the application of modern science—as a form of technology. But technology also refers to an attitude that many have toward contemporary society: "Technology, or science, will solve problems that presently we cannot solve." Although this attitude has some value, it raises questions as well. What are the assumptions on the part of society, the health care profession, and individuals that drive scientific research? What are the principal nontechnological values and assumptions that measure the development and application of today's technologies? As one seeks to create new and better technologies in the area of biomedicine, what underlying assumptions are made?

Some of these assumptions of scientific research are positive—a desire to extend life, to improve the quality of life, to conquer disease, to allow patients to pursue other values that could not be realized if the person suffered from some illness. Pursuing such goals usually results in the pursuit of values cherished by the individual and society. One should recognize, though, that the assumptions are not always positive—the simple desire to do what has not been done, the unconscious assessment of death as an enemy that must be conquered at all costs, the uncritical acceptance of all that science and technology have to offer without careful analysis of the implications of new developments on the person or society.

The careful assessment of a research project must be made in such a way to include a factual or descriptive assessment of what is necessary for the future growth and development of the technology and a careful assessment of the impact of this technology on the values—individual and social—of the future society. How will this technology affect the values of society and the person in the future? Does a society in fact want to change its values based on the possibility of new technologies? Should the technology pursued be limited by the values expressed in the society by individuals? Given the limited resources of education, financial assistance, laboratories, and time, how much does a society wish to expend for the development of new technologies and at what price to existing values and technologies? These descriptive and evaluative values must be explored, but not solely from the consequences desired. The assessment of technology is not an exercise in pure rationality. Considerations about the nature of the person and society, not easily quantifiable, must be at the heart of such discussions.

Discussion

High technology, such as the Jarvik-7 heart, is usually pursued with the aid of government funding and support. Funding for health care and research is not unlimited. Where should money be spent? Does high technology take precedence over primary health care when so many people in this country (and more in the world) do not have access to primary care facilities and preventive care? Granted that there is no guarantee that money spent in this project would automatically revert to other primary care projects if it had not been done, but does it not say something about the health care values pursued by this country? Additionally, since much of the money spent in high technology comes from federal sources, what role should the community have in determining where this money is spent?

Another value question involves suicide, allowing a person to die, and patient autonomy. The decision not to pursue aggressive therapy and to allow oneself or another to die is ethically permissible when treatment is either useless or when prolonging life would cause the patient a serious burden. Is the large motor attachment of the artificial heart considered a burden? Should one, therefore, be allowed to use the "key," shutting off the machine at one's own discretion? Where does one draw the line between suicide and allowing to die in this situation? When a completely implantable heart is perfected, will the refusal to have one's battery recharged be considered suicide? Patient consent is vital both in the experiment involving Dr. Clark and in the "usual" care of any patient by a physician. This is an important part of the patient-physician relationship. Whether "shutting off" the machine is perceived as suicide or allowing to die will affect the physician-patient relationship.

Another value arises from discussion about the quality of life. For the heart patient the quality of life—in the sense of what is valued and desired—is low. The loss of mobility, and changed work and leisure habits that affect one's relationship with the community and one's loved ones, are all perceived as a loss, and rightly so. Ethically speaking, however, this is a descriptive statement about the person's health and not a prescriptive statement about what must be done. If one says that society must pursue some goal—the totally implantable artificial heart—and justifies such a statement with ethically defensible reasons, then one raises critical moral issues. Who gets an artificial heart; how does one choose between the thousands who could use one; who funds such a procedure; is the government responsible for providing this technology to all people who are in need? Ultimately one might pose the question, Is there a point at which, despite a decline in the quality of one's life and health, despite the disease one has, that technological answers are not pursued? Is there a point at which society, the individual, the scientist, and the health care professional say "Enough!"?

Conclusion

There is little doubt that the events in Salt Lake City are significant and promising, but these events also raise thorny ethical questions. Perhaps the primary question of technology remains: Because we can do this, should we do this? The future of health care in its broader perspective depends on the answer to that question.

The Arizona Heart Transplants 59

In early March 1985, Thomas Creighton had four hearts in three days. Two of the hearts were human transplants; one was artificial. Despite the best efforts of the surgical team at the University of Arizona, led by Jack C. Copeland, MD, Creighton died shortly after the transplant of the second human heart. Because the artificial heart used in the surgery (the Phoenix heart) was not approved by the Federal Food and Drug Administration (FDA), and because Dr. Copeland and his team were not approved for research with the artificial heart, there was an aroused reaction on the part of health care professionals, ethicists, and the media. Was the use of the artificial heart ethical? Was it legal? Should Creighton have been given a second human heart even though other candidates were waiting for transplantation? Should the FDA penalize the Copeland team? Although we will not attempt to answer all these questions, a discussion of the Creighton case does offer a background for discussing the role of federal agencies in relation to the ethics of human research and emergency health care.

Principles

If people were perfect, we would not need federal regulatory agencies. But given the evidence of weakness and sin, and such evidence exists even in the field of medical research, society must establish agencies to limit the effects of such weakness and sin.[1] When establishing agencies, however, society must ensure that the agencies do not interfere with or suppress the legitimate actions and goals of people being regulated.

The FDA is responsible for regulating "products that have a direct effect upon human health and welfare and is concerned with the research on and the use of drugs, biologies, medical devices, radiation emitting equipment, food and color additives."[2] In order to protect people who will be research subjects of new drugs or medical devices, the FDA works through institutional review boards (IRB). An IRB monitors the subject's informed consent as well as the scientific worth of the research protocol insofar as it might place the human subject at risk. Approval of test articles is a step-by-step process based on scientific evidence. Although some complain about the time necessary to approve drugs or devices the FDA has a good track record. Unlike other federal agencies, which use the IRB for internal review of research protocols, the FDA sends investigating teams on routine or for-cause inspections.[3]

Wisely, the FDA regulations stipulate explicitly that there may be exceptions to both informed subject consent and IRB approval if, in the investigator's opinion, immediate use of the test article is required "to preserve the life of the subject."[4] If an emergency occurs, the physician or researcher in question must notify the IRB and have the use reviewed later. But the point is clear: The FDA regulations do not exclude legally the lifesaving therapeutic actions that occur in emergencies. Such decisions, however, should also be well-grounded ethically.

What are the ethical norms on which emergency decisions to use a device or unapproved drugs should be based? Clearly, emergency decisions, just as any other medical decisions, should be backed by scientific evidence that the procedure will be beneficial to the patient. As readers of these essays will recall, prolonged biological existence is not automatically beneficial to the patient. Given the patient's condition, will he or she regain creative function, be able to think, love, remember the past, and plan for the future, and relate to family and friends? Will excruciating pain be constant? Will scarce resources be used in the most beneficial manner? These questions and others constitute the basis for an ethical decision concerning routine or emergency medical cases.

Discussion

To date, the media, in reporting on the Creighton case, have not mentioned the possibility of exemption from FDA regulations in emergency cases. Thus the questions about legal penalties for the Copeland surgical team are groundless. When the first human heart transplant failed, the Copeland team acted in accord with the FDA regulations in trying to save Creighton's life.

Whether the Copeland team made an ethically acceptable decision is more difficult to discern. Dr. Copeland said after Mr. Creighton's death, "My conscience is clear," but the painful fact is that many people have a clear conscience although their actions are ethically unsound. What is needed for ethical decisions is a "well-formed" conscience. A well-formed conscience requires that there be scientific evidence that the device in question, given Creighton's condition, had some chance of "saving his life in a beneficial manner." Moreover, some evidence should exist that the rights of other potential transplant patients were not violated. The fact that Creighton died later is irrelevant to the ethical decision made; however, the length of time he had spent on the heart bypass machine, the reasons for his body's rejection of the first heart, the evidence substantiating effectiveness of the Phoenix heart, and, finally, whether one person should receive two human hearts in such a short time are all relevant issues. The Phoenix heart had been used in animal research, and an approved mechanical heart (e.g., the Jarvik heart) was not readily accessible. Thus there was some evidence that the device might save Creighton's life if used as a temporary measure.

The object of reviewing the decisions of the Copeland team is not to second guess but to delineate clearly the ethical issues in order to learn from the past. If the Copeland team had determined that the patient's condition would not tolerate use of the artificial heart, would it have been unethical to disconnect the heart and lung machines and allow Mr. Creighton to die? Not at all. Their decision would have been based on the patient's condition and his future ability to strive for the values of life. This is the basis of ethical decision making.

Conclusion

The Creighton case offers some valuable lessons. First, the FDA's regulations are more enlightened than many realize; second, there is more involved in an ethical decision than merely prolonging physical function. And, most important of all, the Creighton case reflects that ethical decisions must often be made by physicians in emergency situations. Thus physicians must be aware of the ethical norms associated with patient care even before emergencies arise.

1. M. F. Shapiro and R. P. Charnow, "Scientific Misconduct in Investigational Drug Trials," *New England Journal of Medicine* 312(1985): 731-736.
2. John C. Petricciani, "An Overview of FDA, IRBs and Regulations," *Institutional Review Board,* 3(1981): 1ff.
3. *Institutional Review Board,* p. 3.
4. *Federal Register,* "FDA, Protection of Human Subjects," Vol. 46, n. 17, Jan. 27, 1981, p. 8951-89-76.

Mercy Killing and Allowing to Die   60

Roswell Gilbert, 76 years old, is serving a mandatory 25-year sentence at the Avon Park Correctional Institute in Florida for shooting his wife to death on March 4, 1985. Gilbert said he killed his wife of 51 years as "an act of love" to end her suffering from Alzheimer's disease and osteoporosis. Though a jury convicted Gilbert, the governor of Florida has been asked to grant clemency and thus the case is in the news again. Our purpose is not to discuss the merits of the jury decision or give the governor advice. Rather, we shall use the case to compare objectively mercy killing with allowing a patient to die. In other words, we shall question why the killing of a suffering comatose person is any different from a death that results when life-support systems, such as tube feeding or a respirator, are removed from a person in the same condition.

Principles

In order to offer an ethical perspective to the question, we must consider the purpose of medicine. Medicine aims at preventing illness and healing disease so that a person may achieve optimal human functioning in accord with his or her capabilities. But optimal human functioning involves more than physiological function. In order to function humanly, there must be some capacity for cognitive-affective function. If the potential for cognitive-affective function is not present, for example if a person is in an irreversible coma, then applying medical care does not have a purpose. Hence, medical care should be withdrawn once it is determined that it cannot achieve its purpose of improving physiological function so that the cognitive-affective function can be prolonged or restored. The only reason for continuing medical care for a person whose cognitive-affective function has been irreversibly lost is to keep the person comfortable. Even if the family of a person in such a condition asks that aggressive care be continued, the ethical response of the physician would be: "We have done everything possible. It is now time to allow your loved one to die."

If there is no hope that cognitive-affective function will be restored, why not end the person's physiological function and thus terminate life with an injection of air or some other lethal procedure? Why must a family suffer as a loved one slowly and perhaps painfully winds his or her way to a "natural" death? Many ethicists in England and America would opt for this form of treatment maintaining that since the person in question will die anyway, why prolong the suffering? Recall, however, that though the person in an irreversible coma does not have the present or future capability of cognitive-affective function, he or she is still a human being. Though higher human function is impeded the function that remains, namely that of the physiological system, is the function of a *human* physiological system. Thus there are two persuasive and overriding reasons why such persons should not be put to death, even "to end their suffering": (1) respect for human life makes us realize that we are stewards of life, not masters of life. People who believe in God will state that God is the author of life and human beings do not have the right to directly cause the end of their own lives nor the life of another innocent person. Human beings have only the right to prolong life and this only when prolongation will help a person fulfill God's plan. Those who do not believe in God realize that each person must be free from direct killing, else society becomes a jungle. If exceptions are made to this moral precept then the strong and violent dominate and justice and culture are stifled; (2) the second reason for asserting that mercy killing is unethical is more pertinent to health care professionals. If physicians and nurses become associated with killing people, then trust that is the basis of the healing contract will be eroded and slowly disintegrate. If health care professionals offer health care for any primary motivation other than patient benefit, they will soon lose the trust and respect of their patients.

Discussion

Even some who accept the above-mentioned principles would maintain that there is no real difference between allowing a person to die and putting a comatose suffering person to death in order to relieve suffering. Hence they would opt for never removing life-support systems. After all, the argument goes, the outcome is the same in both cases. Moreover, they argue, if one removes a life-prolonging device or therapy from a dying patient, the patient dies as a result of this action. Thus, they maintain, removing the life-prolonging therapy is the cause of death just as in mercy killing the cause of death is the direct intervention on the part of the one who performs the injection or act of violence from which death follows. Though the two actions, mercy killing and allowing to die, are similar in result, they are not the same in process nor in proximate motivation.

In the case of allowing to die, it is true that the patient usually dies upon removal of the life-prolonging mechanisms or therapy, but the cause of death is an existing pathology which is now allowed to have its natural effect. For example, the respirator is removed and the patient dies because of pathology in the cardiopulmonary system. The mechanism or therapy which inhibited the life-threatening pathology being removed because it is no longer useful to cognitive-affective function, the pathology is allowed to have its natural effect. Nature is allowed to take its course. In mercy killing the cause of death is a pathology induced by the mercy killer. The pathology may be induced either by the direct intervention with the natural activity of the patient's physiological system or by withholding some care for that system that should be offered. Thus mercy killing could be accomplished by withholding a needed medicine as well as by a pistol shot. One way or another, then, in mercy killing an act of violence is performed upon the physiology of the person concerned and a pathology is induced. Moreover, at least an implicit motivation for mercy killing is to exercise complete dominion over human life.

Some argue that the ultimate motivation for mercy killing, freeing another from suffering, is enough to justify the action. Thus, they would argue that Roswell Gilbert and others who wish to end suffering should not incur ethical or legal sanctions. Unfortunately, there are many ethicists today who would justify any action as long as the ultimate motivation is good. But this type of thinking abstracts from reality. The actions which lead to fulfilling an ultimate motivation have a motivation of their own which must be justified ethically. For example, though my ultimate motivation may be to raise money to send my children to college, I have no right to obtain this money by robbing widows and orphans.

Conclusion

A final reflection: In determining the objective value or disvalue of any action we realize that the person who performed the action may have been subjectively exonerated from any moral guilt. In the case of Roswell Gilbert and all others in this same situation, we would be more interested in discussing a support system that would have allowed him to bear his sorrow in a more humane manner than in discussing what would be a fitting punishment.

Index

Parents, effects of in vitro
fertilization on, 139
Parenting, surrogate (*See*
Surrogate parenting)
Patient
Bill of Rights of American
Hospital Association,
57
dying, ordinary or
extraordinary means
(*See* Dying patients,
ordinary and
extraordinary means
for)
misunderstanding by, and
informed consent, 51
relationship with physician,
assumptions of, 14-17
telling truth to (*See* Truth
and patient)
treating hopelessly ill,
197-200
Peace on earth, good will
toward some, 94-97
Physician
ethical, 22-25
patient-relationship,
assumptions of, 14-17
responsibility: conflicts
with medical ethics,
7-9
stress in twenty-first
century and, 165-168
effects of, 165
ethics and, 166
lack of communication of,
and truth for patient,
57
at risk for making value
judgments about
patients, 114
Pluralistic society, ethical
issues in, 29-32
Pope Pius XII on autopsy, 84
President's commission on
impaired infants, 178

Problems, ethical, avoidance
of (*See* Ethical
problems, avoidance
of)
Proxy consent, 54-56
advance directives and, 195
decisions of, 54
informed consent and,
differences between
54
presumption regarding
relatives decision on,
55-56
Proxy decisions on Baby Doe
legacy, 183
Psychiatry, ethical issues
within, 90-93
autonomy of patient and,
91
kind of counseling patient
seeks and, 90
patient as integrated
individual and, 91
Psychological research on
behavior control of
debilitated patients
and human
experimentation, 77

Quality of life, 73-76
Baby Doe regulations and,
187
death and, 149
interpretation of meaning of,
73
sanctity and, 73

Readability of forms for
informed consent, 51
Reassignment, sexual (*See*
Sexuality and sexual
reassignment)

CHA is the national service organization of Catholic hospitals and long term care facilities, their sponsoring organizations and systems, and other health related agencies and services operated as Catholic. It is an ecclesial community that participates in the mission of the Catholic Church through its members' ministry of healing. CHA's programs of education and advocacy witness this ministry by providing leadership that is representative of its contituency, both within the Church and within the pluralistic society.

This document represents one more service of The Catholic Health Association of the United States, 4455 Woodson Road, St. Louis, MO 63134 (314)427-2500